The Doctor's PDA and Smartphone Handbook

Mohammad Al-Ubaydli
Director
Idiopathic Solutions
www.mo.md

Online video tutorials by
Chris Paton
Director
New Media Medicine
www.newmediamedicine.com

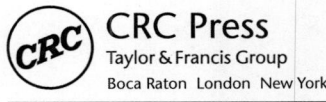

CRC Press
Taylor & Francis Group
Boca Raton London New York

CRC Press is an imprint of the
Taylor & Francis Group, an **informa** business

First published 2006 by Royal Society of Medicine Press Ltd.

Published 2021 by CRC Press
Taylor & Francis Group
6000 Broken Sound Parkway NW, Suite 300
Boca Raton, FL 33487-2742

© 2006 by Taylor & Francis Group, LLC
CRC Press is an imprint of Taylor & Francis Group, an Informa business

The right of Mohammad Al-Abaydli to be identified as author of this work has been asserted by him in accordance with the Copyright, Designs and Patents Act, 1988.

ISBN 13: 978-1-85315-686-1 (pbk)

Visit the Taylor & Francis Web site at
http://www.taylorandfrancis.com

and the CRC Press Web site at
http://www.crcpress.com

British Library Cataloguing in Publication Data
A catalogue record for this book is available from the British Library

Distribution in Europe and Rest of World:
Marston Book Services Ltd

Distribution in the USA and Canada:
Royal Society of Medicine Press Ltd

Distribution in Australia and New Zealand:
Elsevier Australia

Designed and typeset by Phoenix Photosetting, Chatham, Kent

List of contents

About the authors

Mohammad Al-Ubaydli (www.mo.md) wrote the text of this book. He graduated as a doctor from the University of Cambridge in 2000. Since then he has co-founded four startups and is writing his fourth book. In 2003 he wrote "Handheld Computers for Doctors", the world's first textbook about the medical use of handheld computers. In 2005 he created the world first online Continuing Medical Course about handheld computers. He has lectured for the /British Medical Journal/, Stanford University, the Royal College of Physicians of Ireland, University College London and the Royal Society of Medicine. At the latter he has been teaching annually with Dr Chris Paton since 2003. He is now a Visiting Research Fellow at the NCBI (National Center for Biotechnology Information*) in Bethesda, MD, USA.

Chris Paton created the online video tutorials of this book. He is a graduate of Nottingham Medical School and is the Director of New Media Medicine (www.newmediamedicine.com), an online learning and web development company. As well as developing e-learning courses, NMM also creates online medical communities. One of these is Doctors' Gadgets (www.doctorsgadgets.com) a community of doctors and health professionals who use PDAs in their work. DoctorsGadgets.com is also the home of the online tutorials that accompany this book. Chris is also involved in off-line teaching and as well as lecturing on the use of handhelds in medicine, he co-organises with Dr Al-Ubaydli the annual "Handhelds Workshop" at the Royal Society of Medicine.

*The views expressed in this book do not necessarily represent the views of the NCBI or the United States.

About the characters

The improvements we make in our medical practice today are only possible because of the giant advances that our predecessors have made in the past. As a small reminder and tribute, I have named the characters in the book after some of my favourite pioneers.

Introduction – Abu Abdullah Muhammad ibn Battuta (1304 to 1377) was a Moroccan Berber traveller and explorer. Some time between 1304 and 1307 AD he travelled from Morocco to Mecca, and then continued for about 75,000 miles over the length and breadth of the Muslim world, about 44 modern countries. His book, *Rihla* ("Travels"), still gives as complete an account as exists of some parts of the world in the 14th century.

Chapter 1 – Andreas Vesalius (1514 to 1564) was a Belgian anatomist and the author of the first complete textbook on human anatomy: *De Humanis Corporis Fabrica* ("On the workings of the Human Body"). Before this, most of Western understanding of human anatomy rested on the teachings of Galen, over 1400 years old and wrong in many details. After him, the empirical study of human anatomy flourished.

Chapter 2 – John Hunter (1728 to 1793) was a Scottish surgeon regarded as one of the most distinguished scientists of his day. He was an early advocate of the application of rigorous scientific experimentation in medicine. The Royal College of Surgeons of England's Hunterian Museum is well worth a visit to see the artifacts and experiments that he had collected.

Chapter 3 – Edward Jenner (1749 to 1823) was an English country doctor practicing in Gloucestershire, famous for his work introducing the Smallpox vaccine. On May 14, 1796, he tested cowpox, infecting an eight year old boy named James Phipps in the same manner as used in smallpox inoculation, but using material from a cowpox pustule. The boy contracted cowpox, and after six weeks, recovered safely. Jenner then applied the standard smallpox inoculation; the boy was completely unaffected, showing that cowpox had made him immune to smallpox. Jenner called his method vaccination. Jenner was a keen observer of nature and he was one of the first to write about the baby cuckoo's action of pushing the eggs and the young of its host out of the nest so that the baby cuckoo was the only one to receive food from its foster parents. It was for this observation that he was elected a Fellow of the Royal Society in 1789.

Chapter 4 – Jean-Martin Charcot (1825 to 1893) was a French neurologist. He worked and taught at the famous Salpêtrière Hospital for more than thirty years. In 1882, he established a neurology clinic at Salpêtrière, which was the first of its kind in Europe. He was the first to describe Charcot joint, and was one of the first to describe Charcot-Marie-Tooth disease (CMT). But his most enduring work is that on hypnosis and hysteria. Charcot believed that hysteria was a neurological disorder caused by hereditary problems in the nervous system. He used hypnosis to induce a state of hysteria in patients and study the results. This work greatly influenced many of his students, among whom were Sigmund Freud, Joseph Babinski, Pierre Janet and Alfred Binet.

Chapter 5 – Sirs Andrew Huxley (1917 –) and Alan Hodgkin (1914 to 1918) won the 1963 Nobel Prize in Physiology or Medicine for their work on neuron action potentials. As every student of the university is reminded, their most seminal work was done during the summer holiday of their first year at the University of Cambridge.

Chapter 6 – Shibasaburo Kitasato (1853 – 1931), was a Japanese physician and bacteriologist. He was the co-discoverer of the infectious agent of bubonic plague in Hong Kong in 1894, simultaneously with Alexandre Yersin. Initially called /Pasteurella pestis/, the bacillus is now called /Yersinia pestis/. Educated at Kumamoto Medical School and Imperial University, he worked with Robert Koch in Germany (1885-91). With Emil von Behring he was the first to grow the tetanus bacillus in pure culture and developed antitoxins for diphtheria and anthrax.

Chapter 8 – Abu Ali al-Husain ibn Abdallah ibn Sina (980 – 1037), or Avicenna in Latin, was a Persian scientist . At the age of 13 he began to learn medicine and at 16 was treating patients. "The Canon of Medicine", one of the 450 books he wrote, has been called the "the most famous single book in the history of medicine". His writings also covered philosophy, psychology, geology, mathematics, astronomy, and logic.

Chapter 9 – William Osler (1848 – 1919) was born a Canadian to English parents and went on to co-found the USA's Johns Hopkins medical school. He revolutionized the medical curriculum of the United States and Canada, synthesizing the best of the English and German systems, teaching medical students by patients' bedsides.

Chapter 10 – Archi Cochrane (1908 – 1988) marched through London as a medical student carrying a placard that read, "All effective treatments must be free". As the sole medical officer for 20,000 inmates in a German prisoner of war camp — only four people died, three of whom were shot by their guards — he became convinced that the vast majority of illness was self limiting and that medical treatments were generally incidental to recovery. He devoted his work to saving the public from the perils of ineffective interventions. His ideas eventually led to the development of the Cochrane Library database of systematic reviews, the establishment of the UK Cochrane Centre in Oxford and the international Cochrane Collaboration.

Chapter 11 – John Snow (1813 – 1858) was in London during the cholera epidemics of 1849 and 1854. He created his famous map, plotting the location of street water pumps and cholera cases, ending a local epidemic by removing the handle from the infective pump.

Foreword

"Everything should be made simpler but not simple," said Albert Einstein, and PDAs or personal digital assistants are one giant step towards fulfilling Einstein's vision.

Technology is all around us, both in our home lives and in our work as doctors. Wireless networks, broadband connections, and ever-smaller devices ensure that technology will encroach upon every aspect of our lives. This seamless connectivity and portable access to large amounts of information are important developments for doctors.

Medical professionalism is increasingly about being patient-centred and technology offers opportunities to dramatically improve responsiveness to patients' needs. Clearly, any technology brings problems: difficulties with adapting to the new technology, ensuring that the technology works, and maintaining patient confidentiality are just some examples. Instead of shying away from change these are all very good reasons for doctors to familiarise themselves with new technologies to help create a safer, more efficient healthcare system. Technology will continue to play an ever-greater part in our working lives and we should embrace it.

PDAs are a crucial element of this revolution in healthcare. Already doctors can look up results of investigations on handheld devices, check drug dosages and potential drug reactions and interactions, create a task list and other useful databases of clinical information. We can download books, journal articles, and talks and lectures. With increasing emphasis on appraisal and revalidation of doctors, handheld devices can be a valuable aid too collecting evidence to help with professional regulation.

The future, although notoriously difficult to predict, is likely to see us free from being rooted to a particular computer terminal and less dependent on paper based record keeping. Instead we will be roaming with our handheld devices able to make immediate clinical decisions at the bedside or in general practice. We will have access to patient information that will lead us to wonder how we coped in the days of wheeling around a notes trolley and receiving lab results on pieces of paper.

We will beam a task list to the next doctor on duty in a virtual handover that takes milliseconds. A drug history will take moments instead of minutes of fumbling through a bag full of bottles and packets, as we directly access the patient's prescription list from a central database. An evidence-based clinical decision aid will guide us towards the most appropriate investigations and treatment that best suit the specifications of the patient in front of us. We will able to call up the evidence on the prognosis of the particular condition.

The software on our handheld devices will deliver our personal and our team's up to the minute performance information to advise the patient specifically about likely outcome and length of stay. We will immediately be able to work out how many similar patients we have seen, how many similar operations we have performed, and our individual success and failure rates. We will be able to explain how our personal performance information compares with the national average and what that means for the patient. We will be able to record the outcome of each consultation or admission in our personal development plan. Finally, the patient's experience and satisfaction ratings will be automatically added to our evaluation.

All of this immense complexity will be conducted through the simple handheld device or PDA that we carry around with us. The world of doctors is one of information overload. We need help. Technology offers an opportunity for us to access relevant information when we need it, and also offers us ways of managing large quantities of information that we are required to collect.

Mohammad Al-Ubaydli and Chris Paton provide a clear, interactive, and comprehensive guide to PDAs that will help all doctors improve clinical care through an indispensable technology. We need to be well prepared for the many advances in clinical practice that challenge us every day – and this is a good place to begin.

Dr Kamran Abbasi
Editor, JRSM
April 2006

Introduction

What do drug dealers and doctors have in common? From the 1980s onwards, neither professional could do their job without a pager. Only by carrying a pager can a junior doctor leave their ward safe in the knowledge that they will be paged about tasks their patients need. That same junior doctor also feels safer knowing that they can page their senior doctor at any time to get advice and support about the care of those patients. And, of course, the code blue message on pagers is essential for the cardiac arrest team to respond quickly – even when its individual members are dispersed throughout the hospital.

Handheld computers promise an even bigger qualitative contribution to clinical workflow. Not only can you use a handheld computer to do your clinical work faster and better than before, you also can do some things that colleagues without these devices are simply incapable of doing.

What is a handheld computer?

A handheld computer is a computer small enough to hold in your hand or fit into your coat pocket. It is often called a personal digital assistant (PDA). Some handheld computers also have phone features, which allows you to make and receive phone calls – these are called smartphones.

Of all the computer devices created, handheld computers possibly are the most appropriate for clinical practice. While working with information and technology (IT) departments around the UK and US, I heard the same comment from many puzzled computer professionals: "for years, convincing clinicians to adopt computers was a struggle" – yet this changed with the arrival of handheld computers. Doctors regularly buy these devices and use them to improve their patients' care before their hospital's IT department has decided to make the investment. Healthcare computing professionals around the world are delighted that the clinicians now care passionately about computing resources because of PDAs and smartphones.

Several aspects of handheld computers make them well suited to clinical practice. First, of course, is the portability. The devices are small enough to carry everywhere – from ward rounds to patients' homes and from lectures to libraries.

Battery life makes the portability qualitatively different from that of laptops or tablet personal computers (PCs). Most handheld computers can be used over two days of clinical work, while few laptops or tablet PCs can last three hours without requiring recharging.

The efficiency of the battery still supports speed. Laptops and tablet PCs preserve battery life by switching to "standby" or "hibernation" mode after a few minutes without use. The former mode means the computer will take several seconds to respond, while up to a minute's wait is necessary to use a computer that is in hibernation mode. By contrast, a handheld computer instantly works no matter how long it has been since you last used it. This is necessary for the environment of ward rounds, with their continuous interruptions.

Every handheld computer includes a cradle for recharging. The computer sits in the cradle for a couple of hours to recharge completely. The cradle also allows synchronization.

Synchronization is the process of copying everything you have on your handheld computer onto your PC. This means that anything you do on your handheld computer is backed up on your PC the next time you synchronize. Compare this with the process involved in backing up a paper diary.

Synchronization is a two-way process. If you type a new appointment on your PC's diary, the new appointment will appear on your handheld computer the next time you synchronize. And if you write down the details of a test for one of your patients on your handheld computer, the details will appear on your PC the next time you synchronize. This is great for sharing information that you write on your handheld computer and your secretary types on your PC.

Beaming is another way to share information. Line up one handheld computer with another and then beam information between the two. This means that you can send details about your patients to a colleague's device while the two of you discuss the most important points – or simply enjoy your tea.

Handheld computers allow writing. Some can recognize handwriting some of the time, and this is a tremendous achievement given the handwriting of doctors. But the fastest and most reliable way to write is to use a slightly modified alphabet without joining up the letters. This may not be as fast as you can write on paper, but it will be legible, and more than one doctor has noticed an improvement in their writing on paper after using a handheld computer.

The advantage of writing rather than typing is that you can enter information into your handheld computer while standing during the ward round. For prolonged writing, you may prefer to use an unfolding keyboard instead. Unfolded, this is the same size and comfort of a normal keyboard, which allows fast typing in a library or lecture theatre. Folded, it is the same size as your other coat pocket, maintaining portability (and perhaps adding some balance to your gait).

You can enter all sorts of information in your handheld computer. The original devices were named personal digital assistants (PDAs) because of the organizer software included with the device: diary, address book, task list and simple notes. A good rule of thumb is that if you find yourself needing a piece of information more than once, you should take the time to enter it into your handheld computer. The date of an upcoming lecture, the phone number of the manager of your primary care trust, the tasks you must carry out for your patients today and notes from the lecture you attended yesterday will all be useful to refer to in the future.

Extra software allows entry of other information. For example, databases allow surgeons to keep logbooks and general practitioners to maintain their personal development plans. Reference software provides access to the *British National Formulary*, as well as American and German formularies. You can read textbooks from around the world without the burden of bookshelves. And, with the support of a hospital's computer department, doctors on the ward can read x-ray reports as soon as the radiologist types them and blood test results as soon as the pathology laboratory produces them. In fact, computer departments of healthcare institutions around the world are making such investments.

Use of handheld computers around the world

From 2003–04, PubMed lists almost 400 papers that covered handheld computers,[a] and the rate increased in 2005. More significantly, the character of the papers is changing from anecdotal cases and reviews to quantitative trials and sophisticated projects.

At Stanford University, for example, students were provided with handheld computers and teachers used them in tutorials. The teachers would periodically ask questions and the students would select their answers on the handheld computers. The students' aggregated choices would appear on the teacher's computer. The anonymity gave the students the confidence to give answers based on their understanding of the topic, while the results gave the instructors instant feedback about the class's progress.

---

a. The Medical Subject Heading "computers, handheld" is useful for finding these.

Such work is why the medical schools of Harvard University, the University of Cambridge and the National University of Singapore have all provided handheld computers to their students.

Clinical work is also benefiting. At St John's Hospital in Scotland, doctors on ward rounds have access to each patient's admission details, pathology laboratory test results and notes from previous ward rounds, as well as reference documents. Meanwhile, in Lanarkshire, the night-time hospital emergency care team of two nurses and five doctors uses handheld computers to triage all patients and for structured clinical assessments, prescriptions and protocols. The devices generate printed clinical assessments at the bedside and handover registers and reports for the morning teams.

Such work is why Duke University Health System's hospitals in the USA, St Olav's Hospital in Norway and Shin-Kong Wu Ho-Su Memorial Hospital in Taiwan have invested in handheld computers to support patient care. Even without expensive integrated electronic systems, the devices have proved return on investment. This is why Satellife has deployed simple battery-powered handheld computers to collect public health data in Uganda.

About this book

The aim of this book is to help you get similar benefits from your own PDA or smartphone. The first few chapters explain the basics of hand-held computers and showcase how individual doctors can use the devices. Later chapters discuss more advanced uses and issues that you should consider when equipping your team with handheld computers.

For most of the chapters, Dr Chris Paton has created videos to accompany the text and teaching. Next to each set of instructions in the book you will see the 🖉 icon. To see the video, visit the book's website (www.rsmpress.co.uk/bkpda.htm). At the end of each chapter, a clinical vignette places the lessons of the chapter in realistic scenarios.

Of course, the precise details of the scenarios are fictional, but the basis of the book is the teaching that Chris and I give at the annual handhelds workshop (www.handheldsfordoctors.com/rsm) at the Royal Society of Medicine. We hope that the book and videos, like the workshop, will lead to more and better use of handheld computers in healthcare. We know that patients will benefit as the clinical workflow improves.

1

Buying a handheld computer

We can thank the information technology (IT) industry for many things, including falling prices and rising quality. With such blessings, however, come the twin curses of computer jargon and, worse still, marketing departments. This chapter will help you navigate the jargon and marketing claims to find the features you need in a handheld machine at a price that suits you.

Low price is a good thing

Price is worth paying particular attention to. This is not just because saving money is a good thing – but rather that people have a tendency to buy an expensive device on the assumption that it will be better.

More expensive devices do usually have more features, but you may not be in a position to take advantage of those features. For example, wireless internet access sounds wonderful, but if your hospital or practice does not have a wireless network, you simply will not be able to access the internet at work. However, you will still have the disadvantages of reduced battery life and a bulkier device.

Furthermore, the price of the device is not the only cost you have to worry about. Extra software and textbooks usually cost money, and they may be even more important to you than the organizer software that is included with the device. Accessories also may be necessary, particularly unfolding keyboards for medical students.

Finally, if you are buying the devices for your team, budget for training and insurance. You also should consider that cheaper devices usually are simpler to use and so require less training for and commitment from the rest of your team, whose members may not share your enthusiasm for the technology.

For all these reasons you should critically consider costs. For most clinicians, any device that costs more than £100 ($180) should run all the software necessary for clinical work. This is why I advise most doctors to decide how much they would like to spend on a handheld computer before discussing the features. The next decision to make is the operating system of the device.

The operating system

A handheld computer is only as good as the software it runs. The operating system of a handheld computer is the software that determines what other software will run on the device. This includes the medical records and advanced organizer tools that you will need for your clinical work.

For this reason, a choice of a device with the Palm Operating System (Palm OS) or Microsoft's Windows Mobile Pocket PC operating system is essential for most clinicians (Figure 1.1). These handheld computers are called Palm Powered and Pocket PCs, respectively, and only these two groups provide the range of software titles that you need.

Some Palm Powered and Pocket PC devices have telephone capabilities; they are referred to as smartphones. Although expensive, they can run all the software titles you need and mean you do not have to carry a separate phone for your personal calls. You can see the full list of Palm OS devices at www.palmsource.com and Pocket PC devices at www.pocketpc.com.

You should, however, avoid smartphones that run other operating systems. These include the Symbian and Java operating systems used by most phones and encompass many affordable devices. You should even avoid the Windows Mobile-based Smartphone devices, even though their operating system is made by Microsoft. These devices run few clinically relevant software titles. Worse still, few have touchscreens, which means you cannot write on them – instead you must use the nine-button number keypad. This makes entering patient details infuriatingly slow.

The one exception to mention is the BlackBerry device. Such devices are designed for text communication and include a small but affably usable keyboard. They also have a pager-like behaviour for email, which

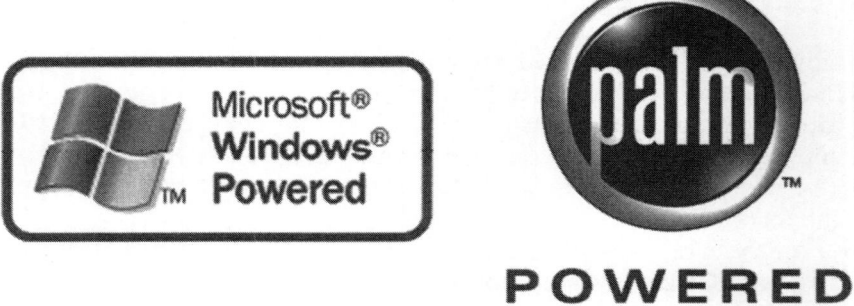

Figure 1.1 Left: logo for devices running the Pocket PC operating system. Right: logo for devices running the Palm operating system.

means that the devices vibrate or ring whenever a new email arrives. Replying to the email is fast and easy.

Not much clinical software is available for Blackberry devices, so the rest of this book will not cover them. However, many doctors who are not working on the wards benefit from the devices. These include clinicians working in public health or those working at the management or policy level. Indeed, it was probably such clinicians who instituted the policy of using BlackBerry devices for all Health and Human Services (HHS) staff in the US. This policy makes sense for the clinician managers in the department, but it is inappropriate for many of the ward-based clinicians at the National Institutes of Health, which is part of HHS. Similarly, Pocket PCs tend to be favoured by IT departments in the UK's National Health Service, because they prefer Microsoft products. For many clinicians, however, the ease of use of Palm OS devices is important and saves money and effort in training and clinical speed.

For this reason, the people who will be using PDAs and smartphones should have a strong input into the operating system that is chosen. Do not leave the decision to your IT department.

The features

Almost any Pocket PC or Palm OS device you buy today will run all the software you need for clinical practice. One feature to insist on is a colour screen – not just because colour diagrams of the anatomy are useful but because black text appears clear and sharp on a white background on colour devices but is on a dark grey background on monochrome devices.

Of the optional features available, perhaps the most universally useful is a camera. This is great, for example, for photographing a skin lesion over the several days between consultant ward rounds. Capturing a lesion at admission also is useful for subsequent case presentations and audits. The quality is not as good as that from a professional digital camera, but it certainly is good enough for a PowerPoint slide. Of course, you should ask for the patient's consent, document the consent in the notes and take steps to maintain confidentiality.

Global Positioning System (GPS) is great for general practitioners. It works with satellites to get the device's current location and with mapping software to show travel routes. For home visits, this provides turn-by-turn directions – even in distant rural locations. This system also is useful for locum doctors who are travelling to new hospitals or practices.

Pocket PC and Palm OS smartphones are expensive but worth considering, especially if you need to buy a phone anyway. The need to carry just one device is convenient, and the smartphones' small keyboards are surprisingly usable and vastly superior to the nine-button keypad of phones for typing text messages.

The one point to look out for in the marketing material is the promise of email and web browsing through the phone, because the cost is still so high. Furthermore, browsing the web on a small screen, although an impressive feat of engineering, is of limited use. In addition, you can carry emails from your PC onto your handheld computer without needing a telephone connection on the PDA.

For different reasons, you should be wary of devices that promise access to the web and email through WiFi. Although you will not need to pay for such access to the internet, your institution will need to have a working WiFi network in place. Unless you have your institution's support, or plan to setup a WiFi network at home, you will simply have the disadvantages of an expensive and bulky device with a short battery life without reaping any of the benefits.

Finally, you should probably avoid gimmicky features such as fingerprint reading. Although it looks good in the shop and may bring admiring stares from your colleagues, the reality is that fingerprint readers can fail. The unreliability can leave you locked out of your device or simply waste time as you try to use it. Resist the sales pitch in the shop.

Where to buy

Shops are full of sales pitches designed to get you buy the most expensive device. Furthermore, traditional shops tend to have higher prices than online stores. You will usually get the best value from retailers such as Amazon (www.amazon.com in the US and www.amazon.co.uk in the UK). ebay (www.ebay.com in the US and www.ebay.co.uk in the UK) is good for second-hand devices. It does sell brand-new devices, but the risk of dealing with ebay's sellers perhaps is only worth it if you enjoy the auction atmosphere of its buying process. Finally, the websites of the companies that make the devices – such as Palm (www.palm.com) and HP (www.hp.com) – tend to be more expensive, although they occasionally have good deals. The one exception is Dell (www.dell.com), which often provides excellent value.

Traditional shops, however, do have a few advantages. First, you have the convenience of buying a device quickly, without waiting for postal delivery. Second, if you are buying several devices in one transaction, you can negotiate a better deal. Finally, you can buy an extended warranty – longer than the manufacturer's standard one-year warranty (only Dell offers through its website). The advantage of an extended warranty is not so much insuring against breakages: electronics today last a reasonably long time and the cost of a brand-new replacement device is low.

Rather, you can avoid having to get budget approval for buying a replacement device or repairing a broken one. It is simply faster to get the budget for a device with insurance at the start.

So, which device should you choose?

Perhaps you are feeling overwhelmed by all the options to consider. Do not worry: other doctors are willing to help. First, many of your colleagues will have devices of their own. Ask them for advice on what to get. It is particularly advantageous to get a similar device to them – at least with the same operating system – to ensure easy beaming between your devices.

You can also get help online. For example, DoctorsGadgets (www.doctorsgadgets.com), the site run by Chris Paton, includes a discussion forum in which doctors give helpful advice. We also maintain a mailing list for attendees of the workshop we run at the Royal Society of Medicine, which also is useful for advice (http://groups.yahoo.com/group/medicalhandhelds/).

At the end of the day, most doctors are delighted with the devices they buy. We hope that this book helps you achieve similar delight.

Clinical vignette of a surgical shopping spree

With one more year left of her surgical training, Dr Vesalius realized that the next year of her career would require greatly improved management skills. She decided to invest in a medium-range handheld computer.

Dr Vesalius searched on Dell's website and found a $300 Pocket PC with a camera, which would be essential for her case presentations. She did not want to spend the money on phone capabilities. Instead, she invested another $200 in a secure digital (SD) card for her textbooks, an unfolding keyboard with which she could write papers and an extra cradle so that she could synchronize at home and at work without needing to carry a cradle with her. Over the next year, she would gradually buy different textbooks at $60 each.

Dr Vesalius's husband, an investment banker, was about to get a Blackberry from his IT department, because he needed the phone and email capabilities. She convinced him to get a Pocket PC with phone capabilities instead. It was not as efficient as a Blackberry device, but it did mean that she could easily beam him shopping lists and her work schedule.

▼ *Cont.*

The beaming meant that Dr Vesalius's colleagues in the department were interested in getting devices. She came up with a plan that provided all the doctors in her team, at all levels, with a handheld computer of their own. She searched online for the cheapest Pocket PC that would satisfy their needs. She printed off the page with the price and presented it at her local Best Buy computer store. Because she was buying 20 devices of the same model in one transaction, the store matched the online price and gave her a discount on their three-year warranty. As she coordinated deployment and support with her IT department and helped train her colleagues, she knew she was practising the management skills that would become essential in the next stage of her career.

2

The diary

The humble diary is one of the most useful applications on your handheld computer. Like a paper diary, you can use it to keep track of your own schedule, but setting up recurring appointments, reminders and alarms is easy and powerful. Synchronizing with a PC means that your secretary can add to and amend your schedule. Extra software such as DualDate allows you to beam your schedule to another handheld computer, such as your partner's machine.

Because of the diary's importance, most handheld computers have a button that takes you straight to the program. This is usually in the bottom left corner. On Pocket PCs, tap on the ![icon] icon and then "Calendar" (Figure 2.1). Alternatively, on Palm Powered machines tap on the ![icon] icon and then the icon labelled "Date Book" (Figure 2.2).

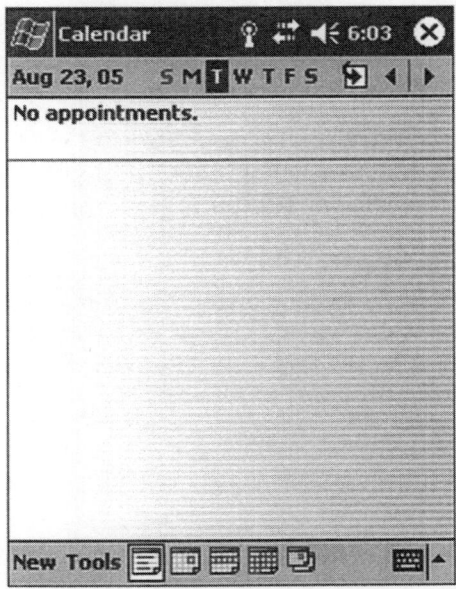

Figure 2.1 The diary software on Pocket PCs is called Calendar.

Aug 23, 05 ◀ S M T W T F S ▶
8:00
9:00
10:00
11:00
12:00
1:00
2:00
3:00
4:00
5:00
6:00
· ···☷☰ (New) (Details) (Go To)

Figure 2.2 The diary software on Palm Powered devices is called Datebook.

Along the top of the diary screen are abbreviations of the days of the week, and you can tap on any of these to show that day's appointments. Tap on the arrows on either side to shift the display by a week.

At the bottom of the screen are the ▣▢▤▣▨ icons on a Pocket PC (see Figure 2.1) and the ■···▦☰ icons on a Palm Powered device (see Figure 2.2). Tap on these switches to show your appointments for the week or month.

Creating appointments

To add a clinic session for this Tuesday morning:
1. Tap on the first "T" in the day selector to get to Tuesday's appointments.
2. Tap on the "New" button.
3. Choose the start time by tapping under "Start Time:" on a Palm Powered device or to the right of "Starts" on a Pocket PC.
4. Choose the end time by tapping under "End Time:" on a Palm Powered device or to the right of "Ends" on a Pocket PC.
5. Tap the "OK" button.
6. Write in "Theatre".

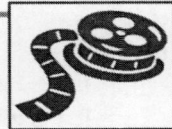

On Palm Powered machines, the "Details" button allows you to set extra options. For example, to make the appointment repeat every Tuesday until the 3 August and ensure an alarm reminder 30 minutes before every session:
1. Tap on the appointment then the "Details" button.
2. Tap the "Alarm" box and write "30" minutes.
3. Tap on "None" next to "Repeat:" and choose "Week" instead.
4. Tap on "No End Date" next to "End on", then "Choose date" and choose 3 August.

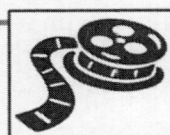

On Pocket PCs:
1. Tap on "Occurs" then "Every Tuesday".
2. Set the reminder to 30 minutes.

Sharing your schedule

Like all software for handheld computers, the diary is backed up on every PC that you synchronize with your handheld computer. If you synchronize with your secretary's PC, for example, your secretary can have access to your schedule, so they can add appointments but avoid slots that you have already filled up. When you next synchronize your handheld computer, your diary will show the new appointments.

You can also use the beaming function to share events from your diary. This is useful for appointments that you have with other colleagues – once you have taken the trouble to enter the information about a lecture that other members of your practice will attend, you can save them from further effort by beaming that appointment to their handheld computers.

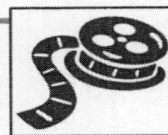

On a Palm Powered machine:
1. Tap on the event.
2. Tap on the 🗐 icon (menu icon) and select "Beam Event" from the "Record" menu.

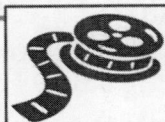

On a Pocket PC:
1. Tap and hold on the appointment.
2. Tap "Beam Appointment".

Make sure that the infrared port on your machine is lined up with the infrared port on your colleague's machine. The screens on both machines will confirm that the information is transferred.

Finally, users of Palm Powered machines should get the freely available DualDate software (www.palmone.com/us/support/dualdate/). This allows you to beam your entire diary to another machine rather than just beaming one event at a time. The other machine displays both diaries side by side. Couples find this particularly useful for coordinating their schedules – for example, identifying times when they will need babysitters.

WeSync provides a more professional version of this software that allows you to keep track of several diaries at the same time (www.wesync.com). This is perfect for house officers who are starting with a firm, as they can know which of their senior colleagues to page at any time.

Adding notes

Every appointment includes a short space in which to write details about the appointment. These include the address of a patient's home or the room number for a lecture.

For lengthier information, however, you need to use the notes feature. On a Pocket PC, this is available through the "Notes" tab of an appointment, while on a Palm Powered machine, it is available through the "Notes" button.

The Notes function is useful for storing the directions to a patient's home or the notes that you took during a lecture. Synchronization means that you can enter these lengthy notes on your PC. With the example of your patient's address, your secretary can copy the directions from www.multimap.co.uk and paste them into the notes of your appointment with your patient. If you synchronize before getting into the car, you will have your instructions for the journey.

Advanced uses

On Palm Powered machines, the "Details" button of an appointment allows you to set an event as "Private". This means that it will be hidden on machines that receive your diary through DualDate or WeSync. With a little more effort, you can also hide it on the PCs with which you synchronize your handheld computer, and your manual will contain advice about this. Practice managers find this particularly useful for creating the out-of-hours timetable. If each GP enters their evening and weekend schedule (as private appointments), the manager can know which slots to try to avoid for the convenience of the GPs.

The security of this privacy feature is quite weak, however, and it should be used only for convenience – not for safeguarding any information about patients. Later chapters will mention better tools for maintaining confidentiality.

Pocket PCs have a category feature. Tap on "Tools" and then "Categories" to assign a category to any appointment. For example, you can create a category for each of the firms that you work on and another for your personal appointments. The latest Plam-Powered devices also have categories which can be accessed through the "Details" button.

Finally, lots of alternatives to your machine's diary software provide even more features. Agendus (www.iambic.com) is excellent for Palm Powered machines, as is Agenda Fusion (www.developerone.com) for Pocket PCs. These allow you colour-code appointments to give you a better at-a-glance view of your day's schedule. They also integrate better with the address book, which can allow you to tie an appointment with the attendees of that appointment.

This last feature has subtle uses. For example, if you remember the date that you met someone from the NHS trust but cannot remember their name, to find the full contact details becomes easy as soon as you find the appointment in your diary. Conversely, if you attended a lecture with your practice colleague but need to get the date of the lecture, viewing your colleague's details in Agendus or Agenda Fusion lists the appointments that you attended together. You can then document the date in your personal development plan.

Clinical vignette of a surgical team

Dr Hunter asked her secretary to enter the firm's theatre session timetable into her Outlook calendar. When she next synchronized, the timetable appeared on her hand-held computer. She made use of this on her new junior house officer's first ward round by beaming each appointment for the next week. The house officer beamed the appointment to other new members of the surgical team.

Because each appointment had been set as repeating, beaming Tuesday's appointment to the house officer meant that the appointment was available for every following Tuesday. And because of the alarm that rang half an hour before each session, the senior house officers were warned when they needed to end their current task and head for theatre.

The alarms also were useful for limiting the duration of meetings. Before a meeting that risked taking too long, Dr Hunter would create an appointment for the end of the meeting and add an alarm that rang audibly 10 minutes before. This gave clear warning to all present and smoothed the way for an amicable exit.

3

The address book

In most hospitals, the personnel on switchboards are extremely busy. This is because so many patients, relatives and hospital staff are trying to reach them to learn the contact details of clinicians. A phone call to the switchboard staff thus means being "on hold" for several minutes.

You can save many minutes each day simply by using your own handheld computer's address book instead of calling the switchboard. But the electronic address book goes further, allowing you to do things that a paper version does not.

Like the diary, the address book's importance means that most handheld computers include a button that takes you straight to the program. This is usually at the bottom left corner, second from the left. Alternatively, on Palm Powered machines, tap on the ▓ icon and then the icon labelled "Address". On Pocket PCs, tap on the ▓ icon and then "Contacts".

The information is listed in two columns: the left column contains the name of each contact and the right shows the best way to contact them – for example, a pager number. Tap on a name to show the full contact details for that person, including their work telephone number, mobile phone number, email address and mailing address.

Creating an address

To add the contact information for your hospital's chief cardiologist:

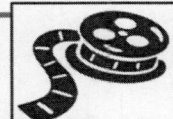

1. Tap on the "New" button.
2. Write the cardiologist's name to the right of "Name". On Palm Powered machines, the name is split into "Last name" and "First name".
3. Tap to the right of other labels to write other information. For example, the "Title" field is useful for noting that the person prefers to be addressed as Ms.
4. When you have entered all the information you want, tap "ok" on a Pocket PC (Figure 3.1) or "Done" on a Palm Powered device (Figure 3.2).

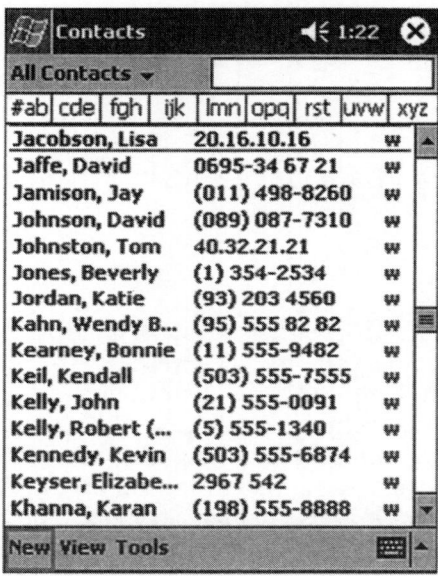

Figure 3.1 Pocket PC's address book

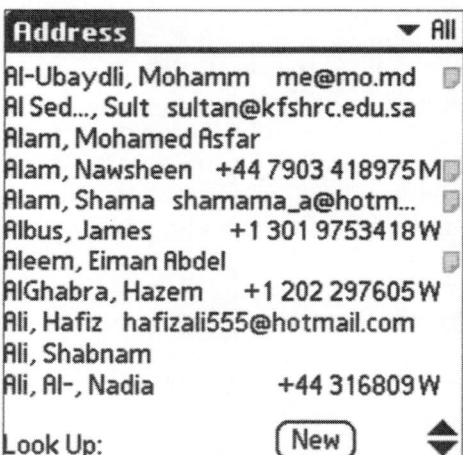

Figure 3.2 Palm Powered device's address book

Categories

Categories allow you to divide your contacts into useful groups. Examples include "Surgical department", "Primary care trust" and "Personal".

To assign a contact to a category, tap on the contact's name and then tap "Edit". On a Palm Powered device:
1. Tap in the top right corner of the screen, which shows the current category, eg "Unfiled".
2. You will see a list of categories: tap on the one you want.
3. If the category you want is not in the list, tap on "Edit Categories..." to add it.

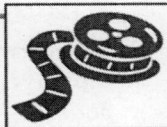

On a Pocket PC:
1. Tap to the right of "Categories".
2. Tick the categories that you would like the contact to belong to. You may tick more than one.
3. If the category you want is not in the list, tap on "Add/Delete" to add it.

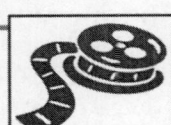

Sharing addresses

You can beam addresses to your colleagues' handheld computers. On a Palm Powered device:
1. Tap on the contact's name.
2. Tap on the 🖼 icon (menu icon) and then select "Beam Address" from the "Record" menu.

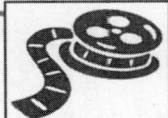

On a Pocket PC:
1. Tap and hold on the contact's name.
2. Tap "Beam Contact...".

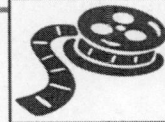

Categories make beaming contacts particularly powerful. To beam all the contacts in the "Surgical department" category on a Palm Powered computer:
1. Tap in the top-right corner of the address book.
2. Tap on "Surgical department".
3. Tap on the 🖼 icon (menu icon).
4. Select "Beam Category".

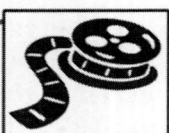

On a Pocket PC:
1. Tap on "All Contacts" in the top-left corner of the address book.
2. Tap on "Surgical department".
3. Tap and drag across the names of all the contacts.
4. Tap on the "Tools" menu then select "Beam Contacts..."

Sharing your own contact details

It is useful to have your own contact details in the address book so that you can beam them. The Business Card feature on Palm Powered devices make this easier. When you press and hold the address book button, the device automatically beams the business card contact details.

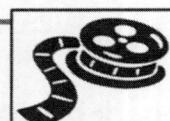

To set up an address as your business card on a Palm Powered device:
1. Tap on the name.
2. Tap on the 🔳 icon (menu icon) and then "Select Business Card...".
3. Tap on the "Yes" button.

If you have a Pocket PC, it is worth paying the $4.95 to get BizBeam (www.twopeaks.com/BizBeam/). This allows you to have two business cards. Put your home contact details on one and your clinic's details on the other. If you press and hold the address button, BizBeam offers you a choice between these two business cards and beams the one you choose. This way, you can beam your personal details to friends and your clinic's details to colleagues and patients.

Adding notes

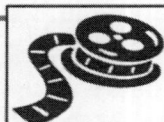

You can add notes to the contact details in your address book. For example, you can include the hours during which a consultant is in theatre, so that you will not disturb them.
The names of the spouse and children of a colleague are wonderful conversation starters...and including their birthdays gets you extra brownie points. To add notes:
1. Tap on the name of the contact.
2. Tap the "Edit" button.
3. Tap on "Notes".

Finding an address

You can find an address by scrolling down the alphabetical list of names in your address book. On Pocket PCs, you can tap on each group of three letters – eg "lmn" – to find contacts whose names start with those letters. Alternatively, you can start writing the name of the contact in the top right-hand corner of the screen. On a Palm Powered device, the writing area is at the bottom of the screen.

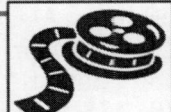

By default, the contacts are sorted by the last name. To change this on a Palm Powered device:
1. Tap on the [icon] icon (menu icon).
2. Tap on "Preferences..." in the "Options" menu.
3. Choose between "Company, Last Name" and "Last Name, First Name".

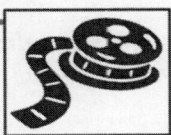

On a Pocket PC:
1. Tap on the "View" menu at the bottom of the screen.
2. Choose between "By Company" and "By Name".

The company option means that it is useful to enter the department that each colleague works in as their "Company". That way, even though most of your colleagues will work in the same hospital, you will be able to see them listed by the hospital department they work in.

You can also limit the list to show only those from one category. On Pocket PCs, tap on "All Contacts" in the top left-hand corner and then tap on the name of the category you want. On Palm Powered devices, tap on the top right-hand corner to get the list.

Finally, the more information you enter in the notes, the more useful the find function becomes. On Palm Powered devices, this is available by tapping the [icon] icon (find icon) in the bottom right corner of the screen, while on Pocket PCs, this is available by tapping [Find] from the [icon] menu (Start menu) in the top left-hand corner.

The find function searches through all the information on your hand-held computer, including the notes in your address book. Thus, it is worth noting how and where you met the person – you are more likely to remember this than you are the person's name, so you can use these details in your search.

Advanced uses

Additional software, such as Agendus (www.iambic.com) for Palm Powered machines and Agenda Fusion (www.developerone.com) for Pocket PCs, adds useful features. Apart from integrating the address book with the diary (see Chapter 3), the software also provides different sorting methods. For example, sorting by "City" is useful for finding consultants in tertiary referral centres. Agendus integrates with maps from Mapopolis (www.mapopolis.com) to provide directions to each address. Agenda Fusion's Power Text feature makes it quicker to enter common appointments with contacts. For example, selecting lunch with the contact "Sally Jones" will create the text "lunch with Sally Jones (01223 558081)", automatically filling the phone number.

Both Agendus and Agenda Fusion can include the date of birth of each contact. The birthdays automatically appear in your diary.

More expensive handheld computers, especially smartphones, include cameras. You can assign a photograph to a contact in your address book, which is useful for jogging your memory about new people you meet. Make sure you include your photo on the business card you beam to others.

Clinical vignette of a general practice

Dr Jenner asked his secretary to enter the team's most useful addresses timetable into his Outlook address book. When he next synchronized, the addresses appeared on his handheld computer. The secretary made sure to categorize the addresses into "Primary care trust", "Hospital" and "Social services". Each clinician's department was entered in the "Company" section to allow Dr Jenner to see the clinicians in each department.

When a new trainee joined the practice, Dr Jenner would beam all three categories to the trainee's handheld computer. Dr Jenner also beamed his personal business card, which included his home contact details, in case the trainee needed help outside of office hours. Dr Jenner had another business card, with his photograph and practice contact details, which he beamed to patients.

Dr Jenner made another category called "Educational". He used this for storing the contact details of doctors whose lectures he attended. He included the biographical information about each lecturer in the notes section. This made it easy for him to search for the lecturer's contact details when he wanted to ask them questions about their area of expertise in the future.

The secretary used a "Patients" category to include the addresses of patients that Dr Jenner had to visit. Of course, she did not store any clinical information about the patient, because the data in the address book is not secured.

She linked each diary appointment with the patient's address book entry, and Dr Jenner synchronized his handheld computer before going on home visits. The Agendus and Mapopolis software provided him with the driving directions to the patient's house.

4

The task list

A good house officer is an organized house officer, and keeping track of the jobs to be done for each patient is arguably the most important skill for a doctor beginning their career. Your handheld computer's task list will not make you organized, but it will provide you with the tools you need to be organized.

Like the diary and address book, the task list's importance means that most handheld computers include a button that takes you straight to the program. This is usually in the bottom right-hand corner, second from the right. Alternatively, on Palm Powered machines, tap on the 🔵 icon and then the icon labelled "To Do List". On Pocket PCs, tap on the 🪟 icon and then "Tasks".

The tasks are given in a list, with a tick box next to each task (Figures 4.1 and 4.2). Tap on a tick box if you have completed its task, and tap again to remove the tick from the box. Tapping on a task allows you to look at the task's related text, priority and due date. The priority and due date are what you really need to manage your tasks for the day.

Creating a task

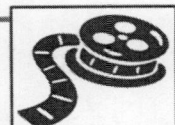

To add a task about setting up a chest computed tomography (CT) scan for a patient with hospital ID ABC123456:
1. Tap on the "New" button on a Palm Powered device or the "New" menu item on a Pocket PC.
2. Write "CT scan ABC123456".
3. On a Pocket PC, tap the "ok" button.

It is important to make the text for each task short yet explanatory. As you look at the list of tasks during the day, you will mostly rely on this writing to give you the information you need at a glance.

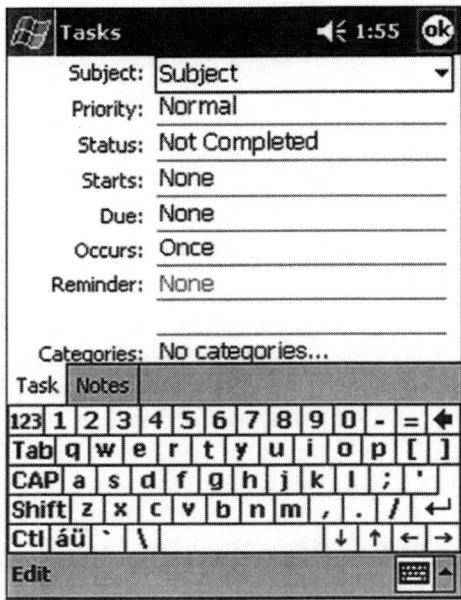

Figure 4.1 Pocket PC's Tasks

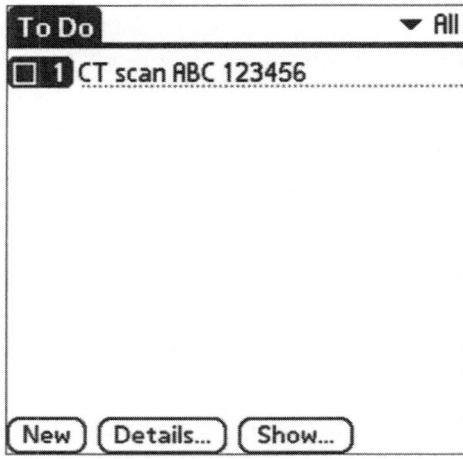

Figure 4.2 Palm Powered device's To Do list

Using the patient's hospital ID rather than their full name is doubly important. First, tasks are not encrypted, so they are not secure enough to include identifying information about your patients. Second, as you fill out the CT request form later on, the ID is the most important detail you will need.

This works fine if you are already in the habit of attaching a sticky label from your patient's notes onto your white coat. Combine this with the hospital number on your task list and you have a convenient system that still maintains confidentiality and complies with data protection rules.

Adding notes to a task

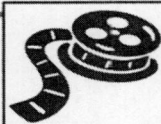

For some tasks, it is necessary to include extra information about the task. In the chest CT example, you might want to include a clinical summary of the patient and the question you want the radiologist to answer. Use the task's notes to do this. On a Pocket PC:
1. Tap on the task you want to edit.
2. Tap the "Edit" menu item.
3. Tap on the "Notes" tab.
4. Write the note.
5. Tap the "ok" button.

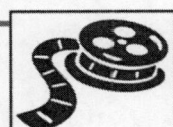

On a Palm Powered device:
1. Tap on the task you want to edit.
2. Tap on the "Details..." button.
3. Tap on the "Note" button.
4. Write your notes.
5. Tap the "Done" button.

Again, remember that the notes part of the tasks list is not encrypted, so you should not include any information that could identify your patients.

Priority and due dates

The key to being organized is to make sure that every task has a priority and a due date. Then you can begin your day's efforts with the tasks that are most important or urgent. Once these are complete, you can focus your attention on the other tasks.

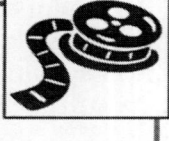

To change the priority and due date on a Pocket PC:
1. Tap on the task to edit it.
2. Tap to the right of "Priority:".
3. Select from "Low", "Normal" and "High". "Normal" is the default, while "High" priority tasks appear with a red exclamation mark in the tasks list.
4. Tap to the right of "Due:"
5. Select the date by which the task needs to be completed.

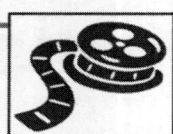

On a Palm Powered device:
1. Tap on the task to edit it.
2. Tap on the "Details..." button.
3. Select from "1" to "5" to the right of "Priority:". "1" is the default and is also the highest priority.
4. Tap to the right of "Due:"
5. Select the date by which the task needs to be completed. You can quickly choose from "Today", "Tomorrow", "One week later" and "No Date" or you can tap on "Choose Date..." to get a calendar from which to choose another date.

Sorting and the satisfaction of purging

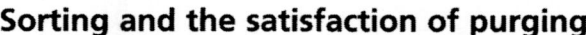

By default, tasks on a Pocket PC are sorted by priority. To change this:
1. Tap on "Sort By" in the top right corner.
2. Select "Due Date" instead.

By default, Palm Powered devices sort first by due date and second by priority. To change this:
1. Tap on the "Show..." button
2. Tap to the right of "Sort by:"
3. Select "Priority, Due Date" to sort first by priority and second by due date.
4. It is worth also unticking the box to the left of "Show Completed Items".
5. Tap the "ok" button.

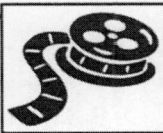

To untick the "Show Completed Items" box is optional but very useful. The result is that whenever you tick a task to signal it has been completed, it will disappear from the list. To do the equivalent on a Pocket PC:
1. Tap on the "Show" menu in the top left corner.
2. Tap on "Active Tasks...".

It is satisfying to see your list of tasks gradually getting shorter during the day as you go about your work.

Categories are particularly helpful for beaming.

Categories

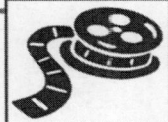

As with the address book, categories are useful. Good categories to create include the names of the wards of your patients and the names of the consultants for whom you work. On a Pocket PC:
1. Tap on the task to edit.
2. Tap the "Edit" menu item.
3. Tap to the right of "Categories:"
4. Tick the box next to each category you want.
5. If you do not find the category you need, tap on the "Add/Delete" tab and add the name of your new category.
6. Tap the "ok" button.

On a Palm Powered device:
1. Tap on the task to edit.
2. Tap on the "Details.." button
3. Tap to the right of "Category:"
4. Select the category you want.
5. If you do not find the category you need, tap on "Edit Categories..." and add the name of your new category.
6. Tap the "OK" button.

Beaming

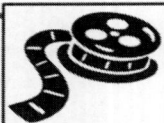

To beam a task on a Pocket PC:
1. Tap and hold on the task.
2. Select "Beam Task..." from the menu that appears.

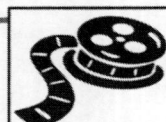

On a Palm Powered device:
1. Tap on the task.
2. Tap on the ⚑ icon (menu icon).
3. Tap on "Beam Item" from the "Record" menu.

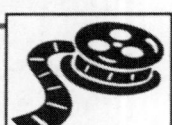

To beam all the tasks within a category on a Pocket PC:
1. Select the category from the list of categories in the top left-hand corner.
2. Tap and hold on the first task in the category.
3. Drag down to the last task in the category. You can tell when all of the tasks in the category are selected because they will switch to white writing over a blue background.
4. Select "Beam Task..." from the "Tools" menu.

On a Palm Powered device:
1. Select the category from the list of categories in the top right corner.
2. Tap on the ⚑ icon (menu icon).
3. Tap on "Beam Category" from the "Record" menu.

Advanced uses

Two types of additional software are available. The first type is useful because it allows you to link a task to a person. For example, you can link each of your referral tasks to the consultant the patient needs to see. When you meet the consultant, their name in the address book will list all the referral tasks for that consultant. You can discuss all the relevant patients with that consultant. Examples of software in this group include Agendus (www.iambic.com) for Palm Powered machines and Agenda Fusion (www.developerone.com) for Pocket PCs.

The second type of software allows hierarchical tasks. For example, the main task for a patient might be setting up a referral to a neurologist, but this would depend on the completion of two other tasks: scheduling a CT scan of the patient's head and putting the radiology report in the notes for the neurologist to use. It is best to set up one task with the title "refer to neurologist" and give it three subsidiary tasks: "CT head", "add CT head report to notes" and "write referral letter". Hierarchical software, such as ThoughtManager (www.handshigh.com) for Palm Powered devices and TreNotes for Pocket PCs (www.fannsoftware. com), allows correct sequencing for the subsidiary tasks and tracks the progress of each of these.

Sadly, no software allows linking to both addresses and hierarchical tasks, so you will have to choose which feature matters to you most. If you are already using Agendus or Agenda Fusion, it is best to stick to it for your tasks. If you end up using ThoughtManager for its note-taking skills (see the next chapter), you should use it for your tasks as well. Otherwise, you should try both types of software, as they include free trial versions that will allow you to decide which best suits your habits.

Clinical vignette of a junior doctor's shift

Tuesday mornings were Dr Charcot's busiest, as they began with her consultant's ward round. During the round, she would keep track of every job for the patients on her handheld computer's task list. From each patient's notes, she attached a sticker to her coat pocket. For each task, she included the patient's hospital number. For the more complex tasks, she added a note with extra information.

Dr Charcot categorized the tasks by the ward on which the patient was present. She also included the priority and due date for each task.

After the round, Dr Charcot carried out the most urgent and highest priority tasks before going for lunch. After lunch, she could go through the other tasks at her leisure. It was satisfying to see her list get shorter as she ticked off each task as completed.

The stickers on Dr Charcot's coat provided her with each patient's identifying information. Combined with the patient number on each task, she could keep track of who needed what without compromising patient confidentiality on her handheld computer.

At the end of Dr Charcot's shift, she would beam the categories with tasks that she had not yet completed to the night shift's junior doctor. The next morning, she would confirm that the junior doctor had completed all the tasks overnight. As Dr Charcot left the hospital, she made use of the "shopping" task list category. She ticked off every item as she went down the supermarket's aisles. Soon it would be time to relax over dinner.

5

Taking notes

Lifelong learning means you will constantly have to make notes, and, of course, your handheld computer will help you with this. The point of the learning, however, is to improve the care you can give your patients. Your handheld computer allows you to access *all* of your notes while you are with any of your patients – something that paper notes, or even a laptop, cannot match.

The software for taking notes is called "Notes" on Pocket PCs and "Memo" on Palm Powered devices. You should avoid the program called "Notes" on Palm Powered devices because it allows only a small amount of text. The writing you will be doing in lectures, from textbooks and during ward rounds is considerable, and you should use only "Memo" for this purpose.

Some handheld computers include a button that takes you straight to note-taking software. This is usually in the bottom right-hand corner. Alternatively, on Palm Powered machines, tap on the █ icon and then the icon labelled "Memo". On Pocket PCs, tap on the █ icon and then "Notes".

Creating a note

To create a note on a Palm Powered device:
1. Tap the "New" button.
2. Write your text.
3. Tap the "Done" button.

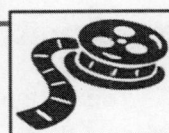

On a Pocket PC:
1. Tap the "New" menu item in the bottom left-hand corner.
2. Write your text.
3. Tap the "ok" button.

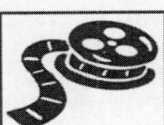

On Pocket PCs, the default is for your writing to be a picture, which is a bad choice in most clinical situations, although it is supposed to be a feature. You will know this is happening because the ✎ icon has a white background and black border. Select the "Recognize" item from the "Tools" menu at the bottom of the screen, and the Pocket PC will attempt to recognize your handwriting (Figure 5.1). It is a nice idea, and many doctors prefer this method of writing because it saves them learning the individual alphabet letters of Pocket PCs.

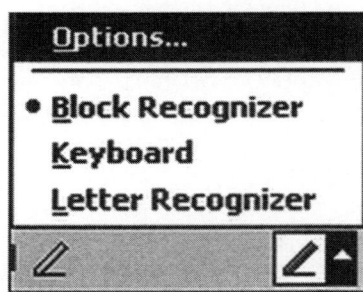

Figure 5.1 Recognizing handwriting

You should, however, avoid this habit. First, because it is common to forget to tap the "Recognize" item, which means that what you wrote will be very difficult to find in the future. Second, because the recognition software is often wrong, especially with medical terms, and can never be as fast as you can be after practising the Pocket PC alphabet. It is worth persisting!

To switch to the alphabet mode, tap on the triangle in the bottom right-hand corner.

Keyboards

As you take extensive notes, you will find that an unfolding keyboard is useful. When folded, it is the size of your handheld computer and will fit into your other coat pocket. Unfolded, it is the size of the normal keyboard of a desktop PC. It can greatly increase your speed and is well worth the investment of $100 or so.

Copying and pasting using the desktop application

Often, the easiest way to take notes is to copy and edit somebody else's text to meet your needs. This text might be from a webpage, PowerPoint slide or Word document on your PC, and, of course, you should ask the original author's permission. First, copy the text:

1. Click and drag the mouse from the start to the end of the text you want to use. The letters you have selected will become white in colour with a black background.
2. From the "Edit" menu, select "Copy".

You can transfer this text from your PC to your handheld computer with the desktop synchronization software – that is, Microsoft Outlook for Pocket PCs and Palm Powered devices or the Palm Desktop if you had chosen this for your Palm Powered device.

In Outlook:
1. Click on the "Notes" icon on the left-hand side.
2. Select "New" from the "File" menu.
3. Select "Paste" from the "Edit" menu. The text you copied will appear.

On the Palm Desktop:
1. Click on the "Memo" icon on the left-hand side.
2. Click on the "New Memo" button.
3. Select "Paste" from the "Edit" menu. The text you copied will appear.

You can now change the text of the note. The new note will appear on your handheld computer when you next synchronize it with your PC.

Finding

The ability to search through all of your notes is what makes your hand-held computer so powerful. On a Palm Powered device, this is available by tapping the ◉ icon (find icon) in the bottom right-hand corner of the screen, while on Pocket PCs this is available by tapping ⊞Find from the ⊞ menu (Start menu) in the top left-hand corner.

This search works only on text – not on drawings. This is why you should avoid the temptation to draw in the "Notes" software of Palm Powered devices or Pocket PCs.

Beaming

To beam a note on a Pocket PC:
1. Tap and hold on the note.
2. Select "Beam File..." from the menu that appears.

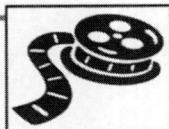

On a Palm Powered device:
1. Tap on the note.
2. Tap on the ▣ icon (menu icon).
3. Tap on "Beam Memo" from the "Record" menu.

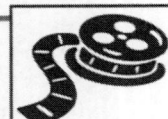

Advanced uses

The default notes software is fast and efficient, but it has limits. For example, you cannot write more than a few screens full of text for each note. You also cannot format text to make it larger or bold.

You have two major alternatives. The first is the word processing software that came with your handheld computer; this is called Word To Go on Palm Powered devices and Pocket Word on Pocket PCs. These allow you much of the power and formatting of Microsoft Word that you are used to on your PC. They also synchronize with Microsoft Word, which means that you can create a Word document on your PC and then view and edit it on your handheld computer – and vice versa.

If you are a heavy user of Word documents, you should consider buying QuickOffice (for Palm Powered devices – www.quickoffice.com) or TextMaker (for Pocket PCs – www.softmaker.com/english/). These offer advanced features like tables and spellchecking.

The second alternative is hierarchical editors – also known as outliner software. To understand the beauty of outlining this, think back to the surgical sieves you used in medical school. It is much easier to learn a list using headings (eg "acquired" and "genetic") and subheadings (eg "infections" and "inflammatory"). ThoughtManager (www.handshigh.com) for Palm Powered devices and PocketThinker for Pocket PCs (www.pocketthinker.com) allow you to write your notes in this way and to include illustrations to accompany your text. They also have desktop versions, so you can still copy and paste from your PC and then synchronize. PocketThinker is particularly good because it integrates with Microsoft Outlook.

Clinical vignette of a medical student

As Huxley Hodgkin began his medical studies, he resolved to store all his notes on his handheld computer. During lectures, he would use his unfolding keyboard to write down everything. He could continue doing this, even when the lights were dimmed for slideshows because of his handheld computer's backlight. The keyboard was also useful in the library. At home, he copied and pasted text from the web onto his PC and then synchronized with his handheld computer.

During ward rounds, Huxley had to write while walking with senior doctors, so he practised to improve his speed. The notes he made were useful to swap with other medical students who had been on different ward rounds. They would share the notes by beaming.

Huxley's ability to search through his notes so quickly and conveniently meant that his note-taking process was active. During supervisions and tutorials, he would constantly check what he was learning against what he had previously noted. Finding a difference meant this was an area he needed to clarify, so he was able to ask intelligent questions to the tutor rather than discovering his error later in the year – or worse still, during his finals.

6

Smartphones

At St Mary's Hospital in London, nine doctors in a surgical team tried using smartphones instead of pagers. As described in their paper,[1] the doctors responded more quickly to calls and had a lower rate of failures to respond. The nurses were pleased, of course, because of the increased efficiency of care. The doctors were also pleased because they had access to textbooks for references from the web for further information. No special infrastructure was needed (the smartphones worked on a standard mobile phone network) and minimal training was enough (the doctors simply had a smartphone one week rather than a pager).

Buying a smartphone

Smartphones are handheld computers that have the ability to make telephone calls. You should stick to those that run the Palm or Pocket PC[a] operating system because of the clinical software available. At the time of writing, Treo devices made by Palm are the best designed, and a version exists for both operating systems (Figure 6.1).

If you do not get a Treo, make sure your device still has a built-in QWERTY keyboard. This is far superior to the 12-button handset of normal phones and allows faster and more prolonged typing compared with handwriting. The trick is to hold the device with both hands and use both thumbs to do the typing.

The network provider will charge the same prices for telephone calls as they do for normal mobile phones, but most providers usually charge a separate price for internet access. Look at this rate carefully, as browsing the web and checking email can end up being expensive.

---

a. It is worth repeating the warning at this point about Microsoft's slightly confusing branding. Windows Mobile for Pocket PC Phone Edition is what you need, while you should avoid Windows Mobile for Smartphone. The latter does not allow writing on the screen, has a small and limited interface, and does not run most of the clinical applications that you need.

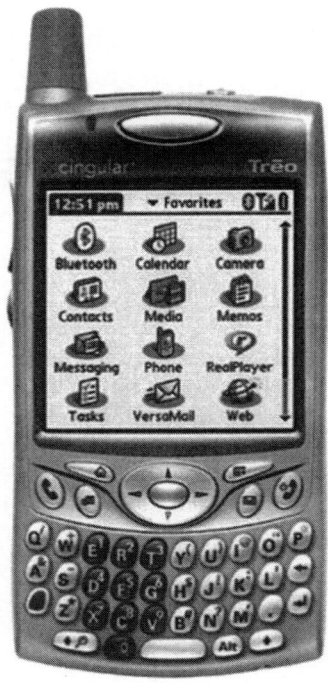

Figure 6.1 Treo smartphone

You can also buy an unlocked device and then buy the telephone contract separately. The device is expensive because its cost is not subsidized by the network provider. When you buy the contract, you will receive a SIM card to insert into the back of the device. As soon as you insert it, the smartphone's phone capabilities work with that network provider.

If you buy SIM cards, you can carry one device for telephone calls but handle billing separately between those for your work – which your institution should pay for – and those that are personal – which you pay for. Ask your institution to pay for the first SIM card and pay for the second card yourself. Furthermore, when you travel abroad, you will also be able to buy a SIM card from a local network provider, so your calls are billed as local – and cheap – rather than at expensive international roaming rates.

Unlocked phones have another important advantage: you know that all the features of the smartphone work. For example, many devices include Bluetooth, which allows you to send information to other handheld computers over a greater range than beaming with infrared. This is great for sending photographs that you took on the built-in camera – especially as it costs nothing. Sadly, mobile network providers often block this feature, because it threatens their ability to charge for photographs sent through their network. Be sure to check about this if you buy a locked device from them.

Smart address books

Using smartphones is safe inside most areas of a hospital. As early as 2004 the UK's Medicines and Healthcare products Regulatory Agency (MHRA) issued guidance[1] that "reason why mobile technology can't be used in designated areas of hospitals where there is little or no risk of interference with critical medical equipment." And a *British Medical Journal* study[2] found that "4% of medical devices suffered from electromagnetic interference from digital mobile phones at a distance of 1 metre. This compared with 41% from emergency services' handsets and 35% from porters' handsets".

This means you can take advantage of integration of the phone functionality with your address book on the wards. After you select an address, press the dialing button on the smartphone. The device will automatically dial the default phone number you have within that address. The integration also works in reverse – when someone calls you, their full details will appear on the screen before you press the button to talk. If you have assigned a photograph to the contact, the photograph will also appear while the phone is ringing.

As the address book is so important to smartphones, it is worth buying software that adds to its features. For example, Tealphone (www.tealpoint.com) is useful for Palm Powered smartphones, because it makes it easy to pick out an address using one thumb on the screen. PhonePlus (www.mesoftware.biz) is similarly useful for Pocket PCs.

Finally, modern Pocket PC devices also have voice recognition. The hardware manufacturer often includes software that allows you to call a contact by saying their name or phone number. If your smartphone does not have this feature Microsoft Voice Command (www.microsoft.com/windowsmobile/downloads/voicecommand) is worth buying. The software also adds several other commands to give to your smartphone through speech.

Similar software exists for Palm Powered smartphones. For example, some Treo devices include a trial version of software from VoiceSignal (www.voicesignal.com); alternatively, you could use VoiceLauncher (www.treoware.com). It is worth testing the trial versions to make sure that the software can interpret your speech and accent.

---

b. http://www.informatics.nhs.uk/cgi-bin/item.cgi?id=801&d=11&h=0&f=0
c. http://bmj.bmjjournals.com/cgi/content/full/326/7387/460

Messages

Most of your colleagues will first realize that a smartphone is better than a normal phone when they see you type text messages on the built-in keyboard. This is faster and simpler than trying to write with the 12 buttons of a phone. Text messages cost little to send and are convenient to receive. You may find that sending a text is enough for most of the occasions when you used to page colleagues to assign them jobs for patients. Furthermore, your colleagues may prefer this method, because it does not interrupt them when they are with other patients.

The built-in keyboard is also good for writing emails, and the email software of modern smartphones allows for comfortable reading of messages. The only question is how to get those emails in and out of the device.

The cheapest and most common way is to synchronize your handheld with your PC. The email software on your handheld computer will pick up the latest messages from your computer's email software and use your computer's connection to the Internet to send the messages you wrote on the handheld computer. As you read and reply to the new messages during the day, the handheld computer saves your replies until the next time you synchronize.

Alternatively, you can use the phone network to send the messages immediately without needing a PC. This is easy, and modern high-speed networks are blissfully fast. Most phone network companies will charge you handsomely for the privilege, however, and your institution is unlikely to cover the cost.

On the other hand, your institution might provide you with a WiFi network. Many smartphones include WiFi capabilities, but if yours does not, you can buy a small card for around $100 to allow this. Once on the WiFi network, you can send and receive emails quickly and free of charge.

Finally, Research In Motion (RIM)'s Blackberry technology is increasingly popular. Rather than having to check for new email, Blackberry-enabled devices immediately notify you when an email arrives, and the Blackberry network quickly delivers your reply. Blackberry devices made by RIM are not appropriate for clinical practice because they cannot run the clinical software you need, but Palm Powered and Pocket PC smartphones can be Blackberry-enabled, which means that you can take advantage of these features. The service itself is expensive, but it is being adopted increasingly by employers, because it increases productivity. Your institution may well already use the service for its upper management staff, so you should ask your IT department to give you an account for your own device.

Browsing the web

The marketing materials of smartphone companies tout the ability to read websites. This is an impressive technical achievement, but two problems exist. First, the screen size of your device limits the legibility of websites. Second, use of the mobile phone network to access the web can be expensive. Newer 3G networks promise high speed browsing and the price using these networks is going down all the time. But a little planning can go a long way.

The most simple solution is AvantGo (www.avantgo.com), which works on all handheld computers – not just smartphones. After installing the software from the website onto your handheld computer, you can choose from its "channels". These include news by the BBC, CNN, Salon.com and the Guardian, professional medical channels like "Medscape Mobile" and "American Medical News" and American and British weather forecasts.

Every time you synchronize your device, the software uses your PC's connection to the Internet to get the latest pages for each channel. You can then read those pages on your handheld computer without needing a connection to the Internet.

Smartphones can perform synchronization relatively quickly through the phone network, and they also allow reading of other websites referenced in the AvantGo channels if you need further information. Most importantly, AvantGo channels are optimized for the small screen and comfortably fit within its width.

If you do not mind paying the mobile phone network fees, the websites of several major companies also are optimized for small screens. Examples include the BBC (www.bbc.co.uk/mobile), which provides the news and weather, Amazon.com (www.amazon.com/access), which provides full access to its shopping catalogue, and *New England Journal of Medicine* (http://handheld.nejm.org/), which provides full access to papers to those with an individual subscription to the paper journal.

Because most websites are not designed in this way,[a] it is essential that you use a web browser that will optimize the sites for you. Devices by Palm include an excellent browser, Palm Web Pro, but you must switch on the optimization feature. Tap on the 🔲 icon (menu icon) and select "Handheld View" from the "Options" menu. Sony devices come with the Netfront browser, which offers a similar feature.

---

a. If your institution's website is not designed with handheld computers in mind, show the following paper to your IT staff:
- Al-Ubaydli M. Principles for designing hospital intranets for handheld computer users. *Vine* 2003;33:88. A free copy is available at www.handheldsfordoctors. com/webdesign.

The Pocket PC web browser, Pocket Internet Explorer, is terrible: it copes poorly with all but the simplest pages and forces you to scroll right and left to read each line of text. Fortunately, good replacements are available. A free and open source version is Mozilla Minimo, which is improving every day (www.mozilla.org/projects/minimo). For around $30, you can get the Pocket PC Netfront browser (www.access.co.jp/english). Finally, Bitstream takes a different approach with its Thunderhawk browser (www.bitstream.com/wireless). For an annual subscription of $50, the company's computers will compress each webpage for your Pocket PC. This allows quick loading of pages and preserves the original layout but with good legibility on the small screen because of the company's font technology. You can zoom in if necessary.

The only detail to mention with Palm Web Pro and Thunderhawk is that both use the computers of their companies to show you the webpage. This means the software should not be used to view confidential clinical details, because a copy of the webpages that contain these details is stored temporarily on computers other than your institution's. Switch off the "Handheld View" on Palm Web Pro and do not use Thunderhawk when reading confidential webpages.

Reading journals on your handheld computer

Different journals allow you to read their papers on your handheld computer in different ways. As mentioned above, the *New England Journal of Medicine* provides free access through any web browser if you have already paid for the paper journal. By contrast, the weekly table of contents of the *British Medical Journal* (http://bmj.bmjjournals.com/handhelds/) is available free of charge to everyone, but you have to register with HighWire Press and install its software.

There is an easier way.

You can use PubMed (www.pubmed.gov) free of charge to browse the abstracts of most medical journals and be alerted to the arrival of new papers from your favourite titles. Most of the time, abstracts are all that you need to read, and your handheld computer will allow you to scan through these and pick out the papers you want to read in full on your PC or in your library. The trick is to use "[ta]" with the title of your journal to get a list of all the papers from that journal (Figure 6.2).

You have three options for PubMed. First, you can set up an alert to be emailed the latest abstracts for that journal. For the *NEJM*:

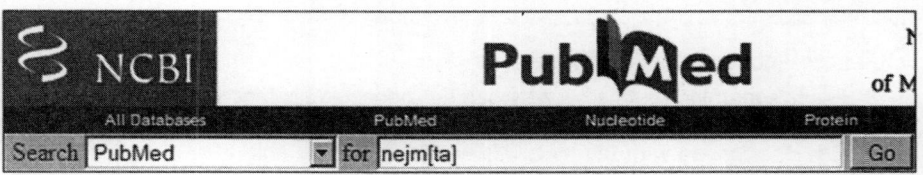

Figure 6.2 Use PubMed (www.pubmed.gov) free of charge to browse abstracts of most medical journals

1. Visit the PubMed homepage by typing "www.pubmed.gov" on your PC's web browser.
2. If you have not already registered with My NCBI, click "Register" and follow the instructions. If you are already registered but are not signed in, click "Sign In" and enter your username and password.
3. Type "nejm[ta]" into the search field to the right of the "Go" button.
4. Click the "Go" button.
5. Click "Save Search" to the right of the "Clear" button.
6. Enter a name for your search – for example "NEJM abstracts".
7. Click the radio button "Yes" to the right of "Would you like to receive e-mail updates of new search results?".
8. To the right of "How often", select how frequently you would like to be told about the new abstracts. For example, "Every" and "Thursday" is a good choice.
9. To the right of "Format", select "Abstract" from the first drop-down list and "Text" from the second.
10. To the right of "Maximum number of items to send" select "100".
11. Click the "OK" button.

The abstracts will be sent to you by email every Thursday morning and will appear on your handheld computer's email software the next time you synchronize.

Your second option is to use one of the National Library of Medicine's free tools to run literature searches on your handheld computer (www.nlm.nih.gov/mobile). PubMed for Handhelds (http://pubmedhh.nlm.nih.gov/nlm) is a website optimized for handheld computer screens. In particular, click on "Read Journal Abstracts", select the journal you would like to read and then click the "Display Abstracts" button.

The third and final option is "MEDLINE Database on Tap" software (http://mdot.nlm.nih.gov/proj/mdot/mdot.php). Running the search "nejm[ta]" will also show you the latest papers from the *NEJM*, and the other search tools can be a quick way to identify useful papers while at the patient's bedside.

Clinical vignette of smartphones

Dr Hwang's morning routine began when he connected his Mac to the Internet and picked up the latest email messages. With the connection still on, he would synchronize his smartphone with the Mac. This way he would be able to read and reply to email messages while taking his bus ride to work, as well as reading the latest news through the BBC's AvantGo channel.

On the wards, Dr Hwang regularly used the smartphone to call his colleagues. Using the ward phones would have been cheaper, but calling a colleague's smartphone meant that he could guarantee reaching them quickly and the voice recognition software on his own smartphone made the dialing process faster. When appropriate, he preferred to send text messages. These were quick to type with the built-in keyboard, took far less time to deliver the message than a phone call and avoided interrupting the person he was calling.

Dr Hwang kept his phone service switched on at all times unless he was inside the coronary care unit. He also made sure that the smartphone was on vibrate mode, so that no ringing when he received a call would disrupt meetings he was attending or intrude on sensitive conversations with his patients.

Dr Hwang had setup PubMed's My NCBI so that it would email him the latest abstracts from his favourite 10 journals every Friday morning. Between 11 am and noon – an hour before the weekly grand round – he would find a quiet place to read the abstracts. He would email the useful ones to his junior doctors with his email software and would pick out a few interesting papers that he wanted to discuss with his fellow consultants after the grand round.

Reference

1. Aziz O, Panesar SS, Netuveli G, *et al*. Handheld computers and the 21st century surgical team: a pilot study. *BMC Med Inform Decis Mak* 2005;5:28. Available at: http://www.biomedcentral. com/1472-6947/5/28 (last accessed 19 November 2005).

7

Choosing extra software

A huge range of software is available for Pocket PC and Palm OS devices. Indeed, many doctors themselves were creating clinical software from the early days of handheld computers. The rest of this book will show you some of the existing tools that you might find useful, but you will have plenty of uses that are unique to your department, family and personal interests.

A good rule of thumb is that whenever you find yourself reaching for a piece of paper to write something down rather than doing the writing on your handheld computer then you probably need some new software. Luckily, many other people will have had the same need as you, so the software is probably available and affordable.

PDA portals

A website that lists other websites is called a web portal. Many web portals cover software for handheld computers – cataloguing the software, organizing it by function and device and handling the payments.

These sites are often your best starting point. Good examples include:

- Handango (www.handango.com), which lists software for most handheld computers and most topics
- PocketGear (www.pocketgear.com), which focuses on Pocket PC devices
- PalmGear (www.palmgear.com), the sister site to Pocketgear, which focuses on Palm Powered devices
- Chris Paton's own site, Doctors' Gadgets (www.doctorsgadgets.com), which provides reviews and news about medical software for both platforms.

These portals provide lots of useful information, including reviews by customers and sales league tables that indicate popularity. The reviews are worth reading, because you can see complaints about software crashes or poor customer service.

The opinions of clinical colleagues can be found on clinical websites such as Doctors' Gadgets, which has thousands of members from around the world. If you are a doctor in the UK or Australia, you should also log into Doctors.net.uk to ask your question in the "Personal Digital Assistants" area of the Forums. MedPDA.net (www.medpda.net) focuses on clinicians who practice in the USA.

Choosing the software

Reviews of most handheld computer software mostly are positive. This is partly because the software is often so good yet reasonably priced. Mainly, though, it is because most companies provide free trial versions of their products, so no one has to spend money on software that turns out to be of poor quality. Do not buy any software until you have used the trial version for a few days and have confirmed that it does what you need it do quickly enough that you will stop reaching for that piece of paper.

A surprising amount of software is available free of charge. Sometimes this is because the company charges for complementary software. For example, MobiPocket Reader allows you to read electronic books and is available free of charge because the company makes money from MobiPocket Publisher, which it sells to publishers so they can create and sell those books. In many cases, however, the software has been provided free of charge by the programmer simply out of goodwill. Many clinicians share their own software, and you should consider sharing your work with your clinical colleagues.

Low (or no) price, however, should not be the only factor in your choice of software. As a busy clinician, you should actively seek out software that saves you time at work and with your patients.

Furthermore, the most valuable portion of your handheld computer is not the cost of the device or the software you bought for it, but the information that you have stored in it. It took you time to enter that information and sometimes it is irreplaceable, for example with data from your audits. You must choose software that you can use with colleagues and that is provided by a company that will survive for at least the next few years.

You should therefore pick software that is close to the industry standard and ideally that stores your information in a format that is used by other software packages. For example, on your PC, Microsoft Word is the industry standard software for word processing. Even if you do not want to spend money on Microsoft Word, you should make sure that the software you choose can store your letters, essays and papers in Microsoft Word format. OpenOffice.org,[a] available free of charge from www.openoffice.org, is an excellent alternative that ensures the availability of your data in the future.

Knowing the standard for handheld computers is a little more difficult, as the technology is newer than for PCs. Sometimes the use of the same standard as your PC is possible. For example, most word processors on handheld computers can open and save Microsoft Word documents, and you should avoid any that do not. Alternatively, knowing the popularity of the software from a portal's league table is a fair indicator. You should use the most popular software unless a feature you need is provided only by alternative software.

Closely related to standards is the availability of the software for both Palm Powered and Pocket PCs. In part, this is an indicator that the company that makes it is healthy and has customers with all sorts of devices, which means that the company is likely to serve your needs in the future. It is also important because it means you can use the software with a device running other operating systems. Even if everyone in your team has the same device with the same operating system, you cannot predict what would happen in a few years' time. You might decide to change some or all of your devices...or someone with a different device might join your team. To ensure a smooth transition, plan ahead and choose such products.

Finally, it is worth picking software that supports beaming. Again, do this even if you are the only person to use the tool, because in the future someone else may get a device and want to share data with you. Furthermore, companies that include beaming in their software tend to be more professional and to have lots of clients. And, of course, beaming is just plain useful. Insist on it with your team.

Searching for software on Handango

To find organizer software that improves the features of your handheld computer, visit Handango (www.handango.com) with your web browser (Figure 7.1).

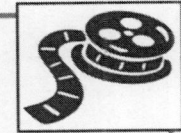

You can search straight away by typing "organizer software" in the space labelled "Search" at the top of the page. More efficient, however, is to browse the entries:

1. Select the manufacturer of your device by clicking on the list labelled "Device Manufacturer" on the left-hand side.
2. Select a device model by clicking on its icon. This will ensure that any software you look at will work on your device. If you cannot see your

device, it might be on another page. Click on one of the numbers at the top to see other pages.

3. Select a category from the left hand side. For example, click on "Productivity" to find organizer software (this is how businessmen think of this software).

4. Select the category that suits you best. For example, if you are most concerned with extra features for your address book, click on "Address Book", while "Calendar" lists software with features for your diary. Software that improves both your diary and address book will be listed under both categories (and several others that overlap), so do not worry too much about choosing between categories.

5. On the left, under "Popular Choices", click on "Products with Trials", so you only see software that lets you try it before buying.

6. By default, the software is listed in order of its sales. If you want a different ordering, click to the right of "Sort by:" and select from the list. For example, "Rating: Descending" shows you the most highly rated software at the top. This is useful, because some free software is of high quality but does not show up in the sales league table.

7. Click on the title of any software that interests you.

8. The top of the page summarizes the software's features, lists its price and shows pictures of the software in action. Further down the page detailed information provided by the developer is given and the reviews of customers are at the bottom.

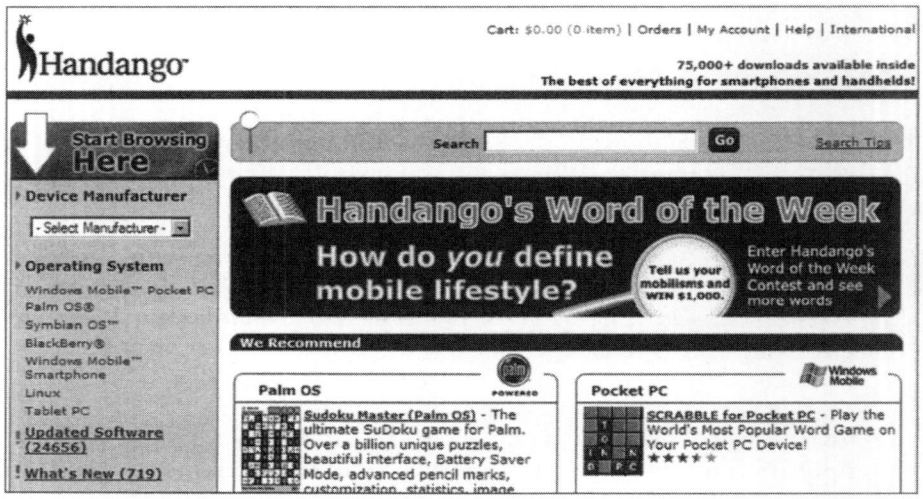

Figure 7.1 Handango's website

A good tip is to note the developer's name. Handango lists this at the top of the page – for example "by Developer One, Inc." for Agenda Fusion – but does not link to the website of the developer. Handango does this because it wants you to buy the software from its own website – not that of the developer. Sometimes, however, the software is available at a lower price at the developer's website and, at the very least, you will find more detailed information about the product. It is worth trying to visit that website by typing the name of developer in Google (www.google.com).

Downloading software

Overall, Handango provides the easiest way to try and buy software.
1. Click on "Download Trial" at the top of the page.
2. Although Handango asks for your email address on the following webpage, you do not need to provide it. Simply press the "Download as Guest" button.
3. After a few seconds, your web browser will show you that the software is being downloaded and ask where you want it to be saved on your PC. If this does not happen, click on "If it doesn't, click here".

Remember where the file is saved, so you can start installing it.

Installing software

The software you download will be one of three types of files. The first, and the most common on Handango, is an installer. It is also the easiest to deal with.

You can tell that you are dealing with an installer because its icon looks like a PC – . On some PCs, the file's name will end with ".exe". Simply click twice on the icon and follow the instructions to complete the installation.

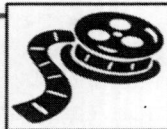

The second type of downloaded file is somewhat common for simple Palm OS software. Its icon looks like a small Palm Powered device – ⬇ – and on some PCs, its name will end with ".prc":
1. Click twice on the icon to start the Quick Install software.
2. Click the "OK" button.
3. Close the Quick Install window.
4. Synchronize your Palm Powered device, and the software will be transferred to it from your PC.

The third type of downloaded file is the most complicated because it is a tightly packaged group of files. First, you have to unpack those files, and then you must manually install the correct subset onto your device. The unpacking process is called unzipping, which is why the icon has a zip running along its side – 📁 – and on some PCs, the file name ends with ".zip".

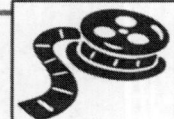

To unzip on a PC with Microsoft Windows:
1. Click twice on the file.
2. Click on "Extract all files" on the left-hand side.
3. Click the "Next" button and follow the instructions until the "Finish" button appears.
4. After you click the "Finish" button, you will see a folder full of the files that you must install.

If your PC has a version of Windows older than XP (for example, Windows 98 or Windows ME), you will need to install the software for unzipping. The best software for this job is 7-zip, which is available free of charge from www.7-zip.org. Download it from the site and install it onto your PC. Then find the file that you had downloaded for installing software onto your device:
1. Click on the file's icon with your right mouse button.
2. Select "Extract files..." from the menu.
3. Click the "OK" button.
4. You will see a folder full of the files that you must install.

The folder usually includes a text file titled "Read Me" or "Install". Read this file for instructions on which files you must install for your device.

This process is a little complicated, but it is as complicated as things get. For the most part, exploring new software on Handango is enjoyable, installing onto your device is simple and, of course, solving your problem by using the new software is satisfying. As you are reading this book, you will most likely be the person on your team who is responsible for testing and identifying useful new software. Your team will thank you for your efforts.

Footnote

b. In fact, this is the software I used to write this book and others. To learn more about how to use such software in your practice, visit www.freedomsoftware.info to have free access to my book "Free Software for Busy People".

8

Medical references

A handheld computer smaller than a paperback can carry the equivalent of several bookshelves of text, and you have whole libraries from which to choose. For many doctors, the ability to carry and refer to their own favourite books on a handheld computer is the best reason for investing in a device.

The investment can be expensive, however, so you should consider your options before buying. The first consideration is storage. Although some devices today can carry a lot of data – measured by the amount of random access memory (RAM)[4] – they still store less than 10% of the storage capacity of the biggest secure digital (SD) card. Furthermore, the cost of storage on an SD card is less than 10% of the cost of a handheld computer's built-in RAM. In other words, it is far better to buy a $200 handheld computer with modest RAM and a $100 high-capacity SD card than to buy a $300 handheld computer with more RAM. Even if you buy a $600 device, you will still not come close to the capacity of the $100 card. This capacity is impressive. A 1GB card can store around 600,000 pages of text. Pictures take up far more space than text, but you will still be able to carry several anatomy textbooks on a 1GB card, along with hours of music and scores of photographs.

The second consideration is that a lot of reference texts are available free of charge, and many are perfectly good for your needs – even if the lack of advertising budget means that they are not as easy to find. Furthermore, for most doctors, the most valuable and important reference texts are generated locally – your own Word documents, your clinic's guidelines, your hospital's protocols or the local government's social services documentation. For around $30, you can create handheld computer versions of all of these and share them with your team.

---

4. If you are familiar with RAM in PCs the fact that RAM is a measure of storage in handheld computers may surprise you because PCs use a hard disk for storage and RAM for memory. However, handheld computers really do use RAM both for storage and memory. This contributes to the speed and responsiveness of handheld computers.

Finally, if you do decide to buy commercial textbooks for your device, consider that each costs at least $60 and many cost much more. Choose carefully and take your time in doing so, because so many excellent offerings are available. It is easy to be tempted by all of these.

Free references

The National Library of Medicine (NLM) in the US makes several resources available free of charge at www.nlm.nih.gov/mobile. These include two versions of the Medline database, described in chapter 7, which allows you to search the medical literature and read abstracts of most modern biomedical papers on your device. The Wireless System for Emergency Responders (WISER) software provides differential diagnoses and treatment guidelines for clinicians who suspect their patients have encountered hazardous materials.

Finally, the NCBI Bookshelf has handheld computer versions of several textbooks (Figure 8.1). These include *Clinical methods* (a comprehensive guide to clinical examination), *Genes and disease* (a primer on many

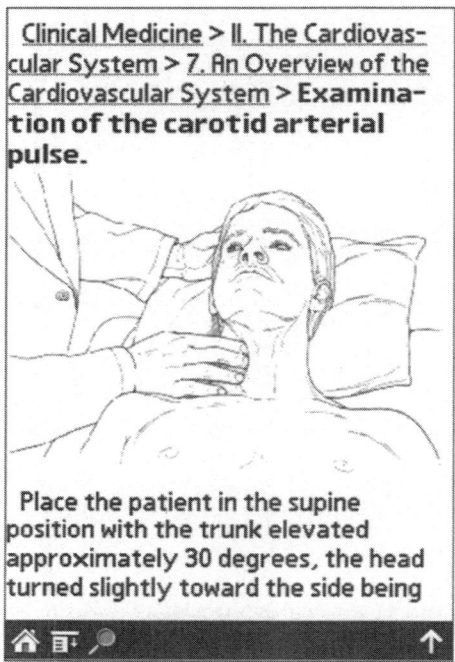

Figure 8.1 Screenshot of the MobiPocket version of the "Clinical Medicine" textbook. The book is available from the NCBI's Bookshelf website.

common hereditary diseases) and *Medical microbiology* (with encyclo-paedic discussions of common microbes). The NLM's own *AHRQ evidence report summaries* is well worth downloading, because it lists protocols for the management of many conditions and even clinicians outside of the US will appreciate the depth of the content.

Textbooks are not the only valuable references – laboratory result normal ranges, Spanish medical dictionaries and lists of medical abbreviation also can be useful. Such information is stored in databases, which is covered in more detail in chapter 11. For now, all you need to know is that the advantage of using a database rather than an electronic book for storing this information is the ability to categorize data and run sophisticated searches. You can find all these data files on portals such as www.handango.com, but if you follow my recommendation to buy the HanDBase database software, you should look through the HanDBase website (www.ddhsoftware.com) in the "Free Downloads" section.

Finally, ePocrates (www.epocrates.com) makes a US formulary, Epocrates Rx, available free of charge (Figure 8.2). The company recently released British, German and Spanish formularies as well. The software's ability to identify drug interactions already has prompted one medical indemnity company to subsidize the purchase price of handheld

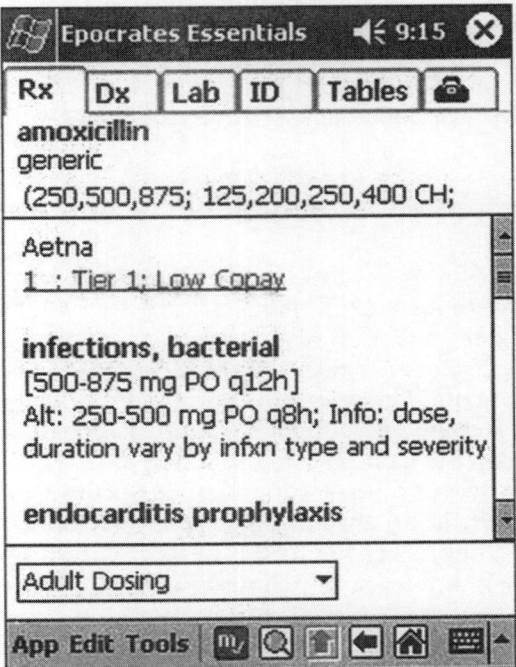

Figure 8.2 Screen from Epocrates Essentials

computers for its residents because it could reduce prescription errors. In many cases, however, the most important references are local ones.

Making your local references available

Your local references are available in several formats, and it is unusual for these to be suitable for the small screen of your handheld computer. Paper is the worst format, of course, because you have to retype the information into your computer before you can use it. Someone somewhere in your institution, however, has the original file from which the paper version was printed. Find that person and ask for that file.

The three most common formats are Microsoft Word documents, Adobe Reader documents and web pages. Each of these has its problems.

Although most devices include software that is compatible with Microsoft Word, the compatibility is not perfect. Ironically, Microsoft's own Pocket Word is rather poor, losing a lot of the formatting that you may depend on to read the text correctly and coping poorly with tables.

Far more significantly, all of these software tools allow the user to edit the Microsoft Word document. This means it is possible for you to write a protocol that includes drug dosages, but for a colleague then to accidentally delete a decimal point in one dosage – worse still, they can beam that incorrect document to other colleagues.

Reference information on handheld computers should not be editable

A great alternative is to use RepliGo's software (www.repligo.com). This comes in two versions: the desktop version costs $30 and can convert your Word documents into uneditable RepliGo documents. Buy one copy for your team. The second version works on handheld computers and can read RepliGo documents. Install it on all of your colleagues' devices, because it is available free of charge.

RepliGo is also good for Adobe Reader documents. These documents cannot be edited, and Adobe makes Adobe Reader software for Palm Powered and Pocket PC devices. The software adjusts poorly to the small screen size, however, which makes for a frustrating experience for the user.

RepliGo's desktop software converts Adobe Reader documents into RepliGo documents. On your handheld computer, you have two options for reading the document. The first is to look at the document as it was originally designed for Adobe Reader, which preserves the layout, columns of text, pictures and tables. This is good for getting an overview of the pages originally designed for printing (Figure 8.3). The second option, which you will find most useful most often, is the text reflow view. By clicking the ▣ button, RepliGo will reflow the text of the page so that it is in just one column the same width as your device. This means you can comfortably read the document from start to finish by pressing the up and down buttons on your device. Adobe Reader, by contrast, can force you to scroll right every few words to read more of the line, as it tries to preserve the original formatting of the page.

To see an example of this, visit www.handheldsfordoctors.com/plos – part of my website, where I store a RepliGo version of *PLoS medicine*. This is the leading open access clinical journal, and its funding means that all its issues are available free of charge. The RepliGo handheld computer version of the issues combines the great illustrations of PLoS with the illuminating text of its authors.

RepliGo is not useful for webpages, however, because useful websites usually are composed of many webpages, with rich links between those pages. A single RepliGo document, by contrast, cannot contain more than one webpage and certainly does not allow linking between webpages. Instead, you should use Plucker (www.plkr.org). As with RepliGo, a desktop version of Plucker creates Plucker documents and a handheld computer version reads them. Unlike RepliGo, both versions are available free of charge, as they are examples of high-quality, open-source software. Plucker is capable of downloading entire websites,

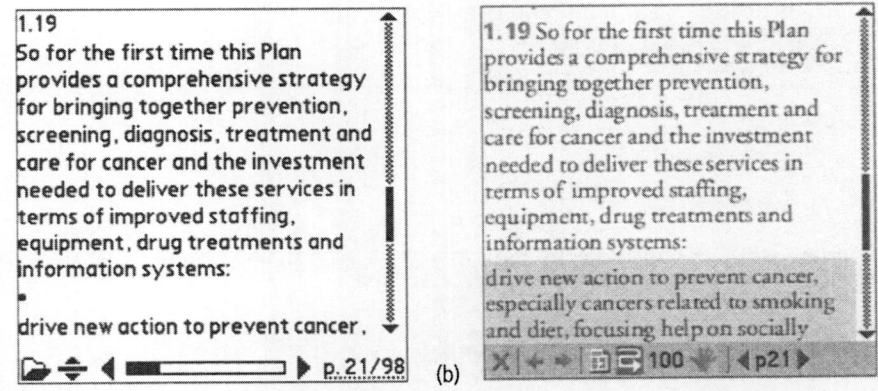

Figure 8.3 Document in Adobe Reader format on a Palm Powered device with Adobe Reader software (a) and the same document converted to RepliGo format and viewed on a Palm Powered device (b)

including your hospital's internal webpages, and compressing the pages for efficient storage on your device but optimizing the presentation for the small screen.

Finally, HanDBase is good for storing local data, such as the appropriate blood tube for each blood test. The software is covered in greater detail in chapter 11.

Converting a document to RepliGo format

After you have installed RepliGo onto your PC and handheld computer, the software can convert any document that can be printed. For example, to convert a Microsoft Word document that details your hospital's protocol for patients with febrile leukaemia:

1. Open the document in Microsoft Word.
2. From the "File" menu, select "Print...".
3. To the right of the printer's "Name:", select "RepliGo" from the drop-down menu (Figure 8.4).
4. Click the "OK" button.
5. Enter the name you want for the document on your handheld computer.
6. Select from the drop-down list to the right of "Location:". "Handheld" means the file will be stored on your device, which means it is fast but will occupy precious space. "SecureDigital (SD) Card" is a little slower, but it is preferable as you have a far bigger storage area.
7. Click the "OK" button.
8. Synchronize your handheld computer.
9. Open RepliGo on the device to read the document.

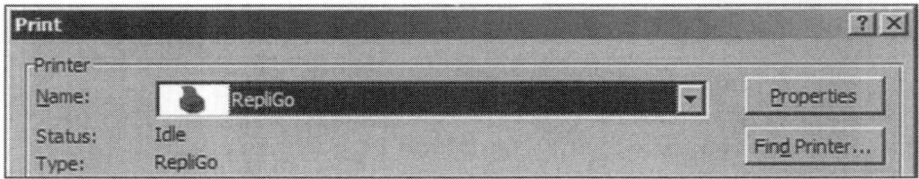

Figure 8.4 To create a RepliGo version of a file you must select "RepliGo" as the printer.

Converting a document to Plucker format

After you have installed Plucker onto your PC and handheld computer, the software can convert any webpage or website into a single file. Your connection to the Internet must be working at the time of conversion, but after that you can read all the webpages on your device without the connection. For example, to convert the website of the government's driving regulations for medical conditions:

1. Use your web browser to go to the main webpage for that website. This will be the starting point for Plucker on your device.
2. Copy the address of that webpage from you web browser.
3. Open Plucker.
4. From the "File" menu select "Add new channel using wizard...".
5. Enter a name for the channel and click the "Next" button.
6. Paste the address you had copied and click the "Next" button.
7. Type a number to the right of "Retrieve linked pages to a depth of". A good number is "2". The higher this is, the less likely that you will miss out a copy of a page from the site, but the much greater the storage space on your handheld computer. Click the "Next" button.
8. Confirm that the channel's content will be sent to your handheld computer and click the "Next" button then the "Finish" button.
9. From the "Update" menu, select "Update all channels" to get the latest copy of the websites.
10. Synchronize your handheld computer.
11. Open Plucker on the device to read the website.

Commercial references

Few commercial textbooks are available for less than $60. High-quality publishers include Skyscape (www.skyscape.com), Franklin (www.franklin.com) and Lippincott Williams & Wilkins (www.lww.com). They make available such famous general textbooks as the *Oxford handbook of clinical medicine*,[1] *Griffith's 5 minute clinical consult*[2] and *Harrison's principles of internal medicine*,[3] as well as excellent texts for each specialty.

You should, however, choose carefully before paying their high prices. In particular, try to install a trial version of any book you are interested in, because this will give you an idea of the complication of the publisher's digital rights management (DRM) software. This is the software that the publisher uses to stop you making copies of its textbook. While it is important to make sure that the publisher does not lose money from piracy, it can punish honest customers. The more complicated the software, the more likely that a problem will arise in the future that stops you from reading a book for which you have paid good money.

Stay away from publishers with complex installation software. One notable exception is MedHand (www.medhand.com). The company sells subscriptions to its textbooks of one year's duration. In return you get four SD cards per year. Each contains the latest version of the *British national formulary*, as well as more than 20 textbooks, including the *Oxford handbook of clinical medicine* and an astonishing anatomical atlas. No installation is necessary – you simply insert a card into your device and it is ready to use. The downside to this is the cost. At the time of writing, one year's subscription cost more than £300. Institutional discounts are available, which is why some hospitals are buying the cards for their clinicians. One irritating aspect is that each card stops working after a certain date. The company explains this by saying that out-of-date prescription information must not be made available, but old paper copies of the *British national formulary* and other formularies still are available in most wards and clinics and are perfectly useful.

That computer technology is used to produce greater restrictions at a greater price than with paper texts is unfortunate. The reverse should be true, and you should direct your money to publishers that understand this best.

Reading for fun

The fondness I had for my first PDA was because the device allowed me to reclaim my reading time. Clinical school meant spending a lot of time in the hospital. I had plenty of spare moments, but few paper books that I could carry. My PDA, however, could store novels and biographies as electronic books, and eventually I would also buy audio books to listen to while walking.

Project Gutenberg (www.gutenberg.org) provides free digital versions of books that are in the public domain. For the most part, this means old texts that are out of copyright, but we all could benefit from a classical education. Each book is available in any of several formats – usually simple text or a single webpage. Use RepliGo or Plucker to convert it into something suitable for your device.

For the latest books, you will have to pay money, and one of the best sites is eReader (www.ereader.com). Each electronic book costs about the same price as the hardback edition on amazon.com. That means a 10–30% discount, but it is still more expensive than the paperback version. The freely available software for reading these books, however, is wonderfully unobtrusive. A lot of thought went into providing a good interface that helps reading.

Most importantly, of all the companies that produce electronic books, this one treats its customers with the greatest respect. To unlock a book, you simply need the name and credit card number of the person who bought the copy in the first place. This simplicity is why I still have the library of 30 books I bought from them and why I recommend the company to colleagues and friends.

Audible (www.audible.com) is the other company that I recommend – this time for audio books. If you sign up for the $15 a month deal, you can get one book and one radio programme per month for your handheld computer, while their $20 deal gets you two books. You can interrupt and restart your subscription whenever you want. Once you get a book, though, it is yours forever – regardless of subscription status – and the company allows you to download it as many times as you want in the future. I have been subscribing on and off since medical school and have gone through several PCs, handheld computers and countries in the process.

I still have access to more than 50 audio books that I bought and can make CD versions to lend to my friends and family. It is not quite as simple as beaming but is still my favourite kind of sharing.

Clinical vignette of medical references

In his prime, Dr Avicenna was a skilled surgeon and an expert in his specialty. He liked to carry around general medical textbooks that he could refer to for knowledge outside his specialty. For £30, he bought Saunders *Pocket essentials of clinical medicine* (www.fleshandbones.com/medicine/ballinger), which included the paperback version and a handheld computer version. He knew that the medical team in the hospital was provided with subscriptions to MedHand, but for his team he just used ePocrates Rx to spot any drug interactions.

Dr Avicenna stored all these books on a $200 4GB SD card that he bought for his smartphone. This card also allowed him to store his entire classical music collection. By connecting a speaker to his device, he could play his favourite symphonies in theatre while operating. For his car, he had a $20 connector from his cassette player to his smartphone. He could play the same music through his car's speaker, but he preferred to listen to audio books from Audible for his morning commute.

Finally, on nights that he had to stay in the hospital, Dr Avicenna appreciated having the books he had bought from eReader. He could switch off the light in his room and yet read comfortably through the brightness of his smartphone's screen. Two minutes after he fell asleep, the screen would switch off, saving the page he had been reading till the next time he wanted to resume the novel.

References

1. Longmore M, Wilkinson I, Rajagopalan S. *Oxford handbook of clinical medicine.* Oxford: Oxford University Press, 2004.
2. Dambro MR. *Griffith's 5-minute Clinical Consult.* Philadelphia, PA: Lippincott Williams & Wilkins, 2005.
3. Kasper DL, et al. *Harrison's principles of internal medicine.* New York: McGraw-Hill Professional, 2004.

9

Security

In 1996, the staff at an English health authority was trained to check for phone fraud. When someone called asking for details about the patient, the staff would ask for the name of the caller and then call back to provide the patient's details. Rather than using the number the caller had given, however, the staff used the phone book to find the correct number. Some 30 enquiries per week turned out to be from callers who were impersonating healthcare workers to get sensitive information about patients.[a]

Fraud attempts are going on all the time – they target your phone staff, your paper notes and, of course, your handheld computer. Worse still, it is easy to leave your device behind for others to steal or simply look through.

Your job is not to figure out all the security holes or deploy the solutions. It is your duty to your patients, however, to take reasonable steps to help protect their privacy. This chapter explains the principles of thinking about security for your handheld computer and provides some guidelines. For small projects this may be all you need, but for large-scale projects that deal with data about lots of patients, you will need the help of your institution's computer professionals.

Only carry what you really need to carry

The easiest way to stop other people accessing sensitive data on your handheld computer is not to have any sensitive data on there at all. For example, useful data for a surgical audit includes the age of each patient, the operation they underwent and its complications, but you do not need the names and dates of birth of the patients. By not including these on your handheld computer, you drastically reduce the security risks. Of course, you can still store the hospital identification numbers to ensure that you can track down individual cases in the future if necessary

---

a. See: Anderson RJ. *Security engineering. A guide to building dependable distributed systems.* New York: Wiley, 2001:167. For the guidelines that Dr Anderson recommends, see Anderson R. Clinical system security: interim guidelines. *BMJ* 1996;312:109–11 (available at http://bmj.bmjjournals.com/cgi/content/full/312/7023/109

When you must carry identifying data about your patients, do this for as few patients as possible. For example, one company that created software for general practitioners boasted of new handheld computer software that could carry the same information as the PC version did. In other words, the handheld computer would be used to store the complete medical records of 20,000 patients. This is certainly useful for home visits...but think of the risks. The PC in your practice is behind locked doors, other members of staff are around to help and when they are not, cameras may well help secure the premises. By contrast, a clinician on a home visit is vulnerable, and losing a handheld computer with the patient details of an entire village is a disaster. It is far better to carry only the details of the few patients you will visit that day. Ask your software provider for this feature and resist their attempts to convince you otherwise.

"Private" does not mean private

The software that comes with your handheld computer is not secure. Even when it claims to be so, it is not secure.

For example, the datebook software on Palm Powered devices has a checkbox titled "Private" for each appointment. When you check this box, the appointment disappears from view. Only when you enter the password does the appointment reappear. Alternatively, the appointment can appear as a grey block, informing your secretary that you are busy at that time but maintaining your privacy as to the exact nature of the appointment (see chapter 3).

It is quite easy, however, to bypass this security. Think of it as a three-digit padlock on your leather suitcase – it does not take much time to guess the code to unlock it, and, besides, it is easy to use a knife to cut through the suitcase and bypass the lock.

Your secretary may lack the computer expertise, and most of your appointments will not be worth the efforts required to bypass the security. However, such password protection is not strong enough to protect patient details and will not be legally defensible in most courts.

Do not use your datebook, address book, task list or notes software to store any identifying data about your patients.

Use encryption software to control access to sensitive data

So what can you use to store such data? Look for "encryption" in the features list of any software you want to use.

Encryption scrambles data into an unintelligible format. The only way to unscramble the data is with a password. Perhaps its earliest use was by an Egyptian scribe in 1900 BC who used non-standard hieroglyphs in an inscription[1] – no vault or lock was necessary to secure those hieroglyphs, only the knowledge to unscramble their meaning.

Today, the military, businesses and healthcare institutions around the world use computer encryption to secure sensitive data. It is powerful yet quick. Of course, as with all security, it can be cracked, but the efforts required are much greater, and the barrier should be comforting to your patients and defensible in courts.

If software does not include encryption, do not use it for sensitive patient information. If encryption is included, make sure you switch it on.

Use password protection software to control access to the whole of your handheld computer

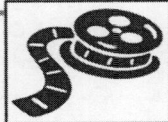

An extra layer of protection is to control access to the whole of your handheld computer. This is nowhere near as strong as encryption, but is a useful addition. On a Pocket PC:
1. Tap on the 🖼 icon.
2. Select "Settings" from the menu.
3. Tap on the "Passwords" icon.
4. Check the box labelled "Prompt if device is unused for" (Figure 9.1).
5. Tap on the list to its right.
6. Choose from the list, including "0 minutes", "2 hours" and "12 hours". The best choice is probably "2 hours", as it means that device will lock itself between your shifts but not during your work day.
7. You can have a "Simple 4 digit password" or a "Strong alphanumeric password". As you will have encryption for patient data, it is best to just tap on "Simple 4 digit password". The advantage of this is that you can quickly tap it using the large buttons on the screen – even using your thumb.
8. Tap the four digits you want for your password.
9. Tap the "ENTER" button.

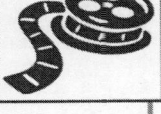

On a Palm Powered device:
1. Tap on the 🖼 icon.
2. Make sure the top-right corner shows "All". If not, tap on the triangle and select "All" from the list of categories.
3. Tap on the "Security" icon.
4. Under "Password:" (Figure 9.2) is a rectangle labelled "-Unassigned-" (if the password has not yet been assigned) or "-Assigned-" (if it has). Tap on the rectangle.
5. Under "Enter a password:", enter your password.
6. Under "Hint:", you can write some text to remind you of the password in case you forget it.

▼ Cont.

7. Click the "OK" button, re-enter your password to confirm it, and click the "OK" button again.
8. Tap on the rectangle under "Auto Lock Handheld:". You will be prompted to enter your password.
9. The choices available are "Never" (the device never automatically locks itself), "On power off" (it locks itself whenever the screen is off, meaning you will have to enter the password the next time you try to use the device), "At a preset time", and "After a preset delay". Tap on the choice you want and follow the instructions.
10. Tap the "OK" button.
11. At any time that you want to lock your device you can tap the "Lock & Turn Off..." button. Otherwise, the device will lock itself automatically according to the setting you chose.

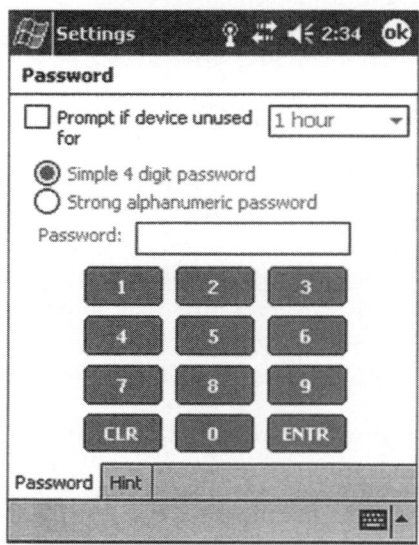

Figure 9.1 Enabling password protection for your Pocket PC

"At a preset time" is a good choice, especially with a time like 2 am. This means that the device will lock itself shortly after midnight, when you usually will be asleep, and will require you to unlock it at the start of your shift the next morning.

When you share data, you must share security

When you synchronize your handheld computer with a PC, all its data is copied onto the PC. If the data is not encrypted on your handheld com-

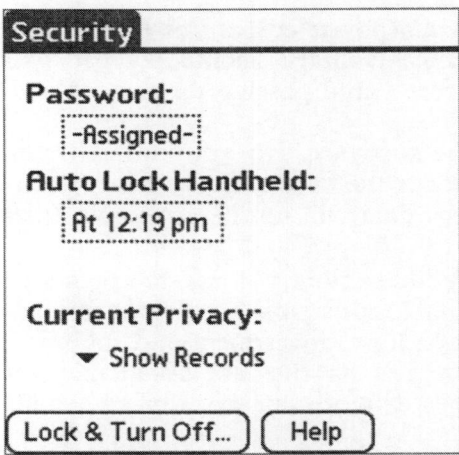

Figure 9.2 Enabling password protection for your Palm Powered device

puter, it will not be encrypted on the PC. To gain access to unencrypted data on a PC is even easier than doing so on your device. Again, make sure you use encryption.

You should also secure the PC itself. For example, make sure a password is required to access your PC's files. It is also a good idea not to synchronize with too many PCs: it is useful to synchronize with your work PC and your home PC, and perhaps your secretary's PC as well, but any more than that is probably too many for you to manage security.

The same principle applies to beaming data. When you beam patient details to another handheld computer, you must make sure that the user of that device understands the importance of encryption and passwords. It is relatively easy to turn off encryption, and many users do so to avoid the inconvenience of having to enter the password to access clinical data. You must explain to other members of the team that it is their ethical and legal duty to take good care of data on their device. If a colleague does not want to or does not know how to stick to these practices, do not beam them the data.

Advanced uses

Extra software can help with encryption. For example, eWallet (www.iliumsoft.com) provides fast and safe encryption of your credit card details, website passwords and personal health information. The software described in the next two chapters includes encryption for safe storage of your patient's information.

Other software improves the automatic locking of your handheld computer. Examples include SafeGuard PDA for Pocket PCs (www.utimaco.

com) and TealLock Corporate edition for Palm Powered devices (www. tealpoint.com). Their advantages include keypad passwords – even for Palm Powered devices – and passwords longer than four digits – even on Pocket PCs.

Furthermore, the software can automatically encrypt data at the same time that it locks the device. Be careful with this feature though, because it means the data will not be accessible when you synchronize with your PC.

Finally, a considerable amount of risk can be mitigated if your device does not store the data, but simply accesses it through your institution's network. This takes a lot of investment and support from your local IT department, but it means that the data is available whenever your device is on the institution's network but stops being available when you take your device home.

Clinical vignette of a pathologist

Dr Osler changed the password on his PC every three months. His hospital's IT department had requested this for all work PCs, but Dr Osler carried the habit to his home PC. He did this because he synchronized his Pocket PC with both PCs, so he knew that he needed to secure his home PC as well as the one at the office.

Dr Osler also made sure he used different passwords for all the websites he needed to access. He bought eWallet for his handheld computer and installed the desktop version on his home and work PCs. After he entered the password on his PC, eWallet would automatically fill out the passwords for the different websites he needed to visit. While away from his PCs, the handheld computer version of eWallet provided his full credit card details, as well as his wife's, and all the other administrative details he would need to fill out forms during the day. All this data was safe because eWallet encrypts it.

Dr Osler also bought SafeGuard PDA, so he could use a six-digit pin number to lock his Pocket PC. The device would lock after four hours without use.

Dr Osler also used the software to encrypt a folder on his device that contained photographs of pathology specimens. The photographs were useful for tutorials with his students and colleagues. However, because he also wanted to store Word documents in the folder with details about the patient to which each photograph belonged, he needed to encrypt the folder. This meant that the photographs and Word documents were not readable on his home and work PCs or on his secretary's PC, which protected his patients' privacy.

Reference

1. Kahn D. *The codebreakers*. Macmillan, 1967

10

Databases

A database is the computer equivalent of a filing cabinet full of forms. Like a filing cabinet, a database can store a lot of information, and by using forms, the information is structured, which paves the way for statistical analysis and audits.

A database on a handheld computer has many advantages over a filing cabinet. First, you can carry all the forms you need. This is great for audits, because you can enter data about patients at any time, including while you are with the patient during the ward round or when you can get hold of the patient's notes from the consultant's secretary.

Second, you can carry all the information you have filled out in the past. Not only is the handheld device orders of magnitude smaller than a filing cabinet, the sorting and searching tools are very fast. For example, if you have a list of patients, it only takes a few seconds to sort it by each patient's name and then to sort it again by consultant's name. You can quickly search for a patient whose date of birth is before a certain year and whose blood results are within a certain range.

Finally, you can share the information with colleagues. Beaming makes this quick and easy to do as you meet with colleagues during the day. It takes more effort and expertise to do this with synchronization, but it means you can get the information without needing a face-to-face meeting.

Choice of database

Many database programs are available to choose from. For the Palm Powered devices, you can use Pilot-DB (http://pilot-db.sourceforge.net/), which is free of charge but lacks encryption and is not very user friendly. JFile is well worth the $25 (www.land-j.com), as is Sprint DB Pro for Pocket PCs (www.kaione.com).

For most users, however, HanDBase is the most appropriate database software. First, it is available for both Palm Powered and Pocket PC devices, which makes sharing data with your colleagues easier. Second, it has the most example databases available, both free of charge and for sale, which means that you can use someone else's work rather than design your own database forms.

Using someone else's database

Freshly installed database software has no forms for you to enter data, so you must either spend the time creating your own forms or use someone else's. Many doctors prefer creating a form that is perfectly suited to their habits and work, and this has its advantages. For the novice user, however, creating a form can be daunting. Furthermore, it is more efficient to use someone else's work and customize it than to create a brand new form. Finally, standardization can be a good thing, especially if you would like to share data with colleagues. In other words, if you use a different form to your colleagues, you cannot share the data in each other's forms.

This is why so many medical institutions make database forms available to their members. For example, the Association of Surgeons of Great Britain and Ireland (www.asgbi.org.uk) has created a surgical logbook built on HanDBase, which you can download free of charge from www. surgeonslog.com. What is particularly impressive is the ability to transfer the data from your handheld computer to the association's website so you can back up and view it over the web.

The Royal College of Anaesthetists' logbook is available at www. logbook.org.uk and is also built on HanDBase. My own website (www. handheldsfordoctors.com/databases) makes other databases that you can customize and share with colleagues available free of charge. The next few examples will use the surgical logbook HanDBase database from this site.

Entering data

To open HanDBase on Pocket PCs, tap on the ▨ icon, then "Program Files" and then the icon labelled "HanDBase". On Palm Powered machines, tap on the ▨ icon and then the icon labelled "HanDBase". You will see a list of the databases you have installed. Tap on "Surgical logbook" for this example (Figure 10.1).

HanDBase
All
Choose Database:
Surgical logbook
New
Open
Beam
Tools
Details

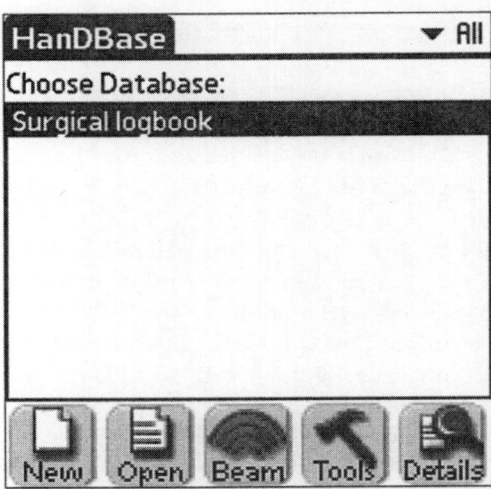

Figure 10.1 HanDBase lists the databases you have installed

For security, this database is encrypted. The default password is blank, so just tap the "OK" button, but you will have to change this when you finish entering data.

You will see a list of column headings across the top, including "ID", "Date", "Patient ID", "DOB", "Sex" and "Age". As you add data about your operations, a row will appear for each operation.

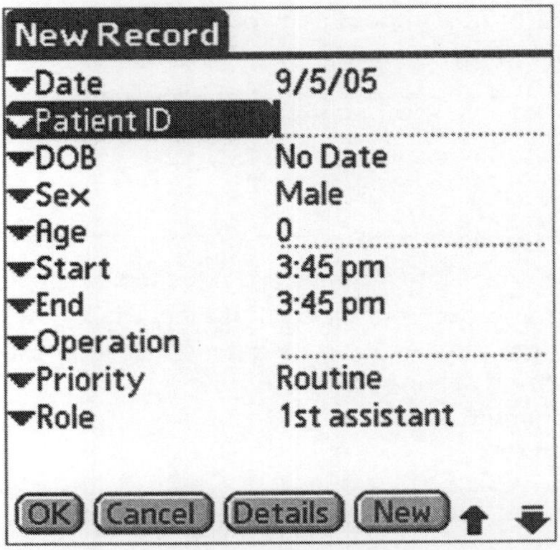

New Record
Date 9/5/05
Patient ID
DOB No Date
Sex Male
Age 0
Start 3:45 pm
End 3:45 pm
Operation
Priority Routine
Role 1st assistant
OK
Cancel
Details
New

Figure 10.2 Tap the "New" button to enter a record in your database. This example is from the surgical logbook database.

To enter data:

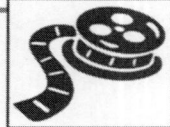

1. Tap the "New" button.
2. By default, the date of the operation is today's date. Tap to the right of "Date" to select a different one.
3. Write the patient's hospital identification number to the right of "Patient ID".
4. Tap to the right of "DOB" to select the patient's date of birth.
5. Select the patient's sex by tapping to the right of "Sex".
6. Write the patient's age to the right of "Age".
7. By default, the current time is used for the operation's starting and ending times. Tap to the right of "Start" and "End" to select different times.
8. Tap on "Operation" to select the operation from the list of operations. If the operation you want is not in the list, tap "Edit Popup List" to add its name.
9. By default, the priority is "Routine". Tap on "Priority" to select an alternative, such as "Day case", "Emergency" or "Urgent".
10. By default, your role is "1st assistant". Tap on "Role" to select a different one, such as "Performed alone".
11. This should be enough information to enter about the patient at the start. It is useful for your own records and for submission to your surgical college, however, to enter more information. For example, further down the form, you can document the patient's past medical history (tap to the right of "PMH") and complications at 24 hours, one month and in the long term.
12. Tap on the ⬇ button to go down and the ⬆ button to go up.
13. When you are finished, tap the "OK" button.

Sorting

In each database, the records usually are listed in the order you entered them. To choose a different method, tap on a column name. For example, to sort by date, with the latest operations appearing at the top:

1. Tap on the column titled "Date".
2. Tap "Sort Reverse".

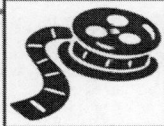

You can sort using multiple criteria. For example, to sort your operations first by your role and then by the date of the operation:
1. Tap on the "Tools" button.
2. Tap on the "Sort" button.
3. Tap to the right of "Primary Sort:" and select "Role".
4. Tap to the right of "Secondary Sort:" and select "Date".
5. Underneath "Secondary Sort:", tap on "Reverse".
6. Tap the "OK" button.

Filtering

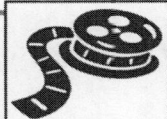

Filtering allows you to find a particular group of patients. For example, to find all the patients between the age of 30 and 40 years who had diabetes in their past medical history:
1. Tap on the "Tools" button.
2. Tap on the "Filter" button.
3. Tick the box labelled "Filter 1 Enabled".
4. Tap to the right of "Select Field:" and select "Age".
5. Write "30" to right of "Lower Limit:" and "40" to the right of "Upper Limit:".
6. Tick the box labelled "Filter 2 Enabled".
7. Tap to the right of "Select Field:" and select "PMH".
8. Write "diabetes" to the right of "Must Contain:".
9. Tap on the ▼ button to go down and the ▲ button to go up and add any other filters.
10. When you are finished, tap the "OK" button.

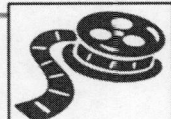

The list of operations now will include only those that meet the criteria of these filters.
To remove the filter:
1. Tap on the "Tools" button.
2. Tap on the "Filter" button.
3. Untick the boxes labelled "Filter 1 Enabled" and "Filter 2 Enabled".
4. Tap the "OK" button.

The list will return to showing all of the operations.

Running a report

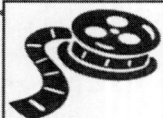

You can do simple statistical analyses of your data. To find the average age of your patients on a Palm Powered device, tap on the [i] icon (menu icon). Then, on this device or a Pocket PC:

1. Tap on the "Actions" menu and select "Run Report".
2. Tap on "Select Field".
3. Tap on "Age".
4. Tap the "Go" button.

You will see the average age to the right of "Average:", as well as the minimum ("Min value:") and maximum ("Max value:") ages. The "Sum" is not useful in this case, but it would be important for adding up the cost column in a database that tracked the purchases made by your department.

Designing a database

It is technically fairly easy to design your own database, but coming up with a good design can be hard. It certainly takes experience and a little thinking in advance. It is worth trying the example databases with your patients for a few days to note which parts of the design you would like to change.

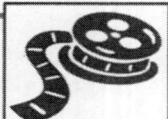

To change the design of an existing database on your Pocket PCs, tap on the [■] icon, then on "Program Files" and then on the icon labelled "HanDBase". On a Palm Powered device, tap on the [●] icon and then the icon labelled "HanDBase". Then:

1. Tap on the name of the database you want to edit.
2. Tap on the "Details" button.
3. If the database is encrypted or password protected, enter the password and tap the "OK" button.
4. Tap on the "Fields" button.

You will see a list of fields. Each field is the equivalent of a column heading that you see when listing the records in your database. Tap on the field that you want to edit. For example, if you tap on "DOB" from the surgical logbook database, you can see that its "Field Type:" is "Date" (Figure 10.3). This means that changing the value of this date in a record will bring up a calendar.

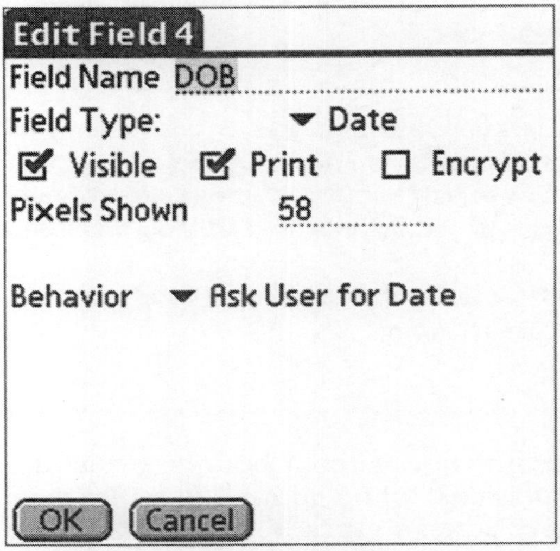

Figure 10.3 The date of birth field in HanDBase

If you had selected "Text" instead, you would have to write "01/26/1976" for a patient whose date of birth is 26 January 1976. This might seem faster, but it means that running the filters feature is practically useless for "DOB". You will not be able to filter patients born before 1975, for example, as the database does not treat "DOB" as a date.

Similarly, the "Age" field is an "Integer", which means that the database treats it as a whole number. This is useful because the surgical logbook database will prevent you writing "67.5" or "67a" by mistake, which keeps your data clean. It also means you can see the sum of that field's data when you run a report on the database.

As you can see, designing a database can be complicated at the start. Fortunately, HanDBase's website has excellent explanations of all of the field types, as well as excellent tutorials that walk you through setting up your own database (www.ddhsoftware.com/support.html). The RSM course that we run every year (www.handheldsfordoctors.com/rsm) also provides hands-on training.

Advanced uses

You can share data between databases. To beam from your Pocket PCs, tap on the 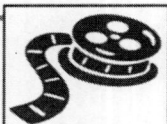 icon, then on "Program Files" and then on the icon labelled "HanDBase". On a Palm Powered device, tap on the ⬤ and then the icon labelled "HanDBase". Then:

1. Tap on the database you would like to beam.
2. Tap on the "Beam" button.
3. Tap on "IR".

To share the information without beaming, you will need the help of a computer professional who will need to set up your institution's network. If you have access to such a professional, it is worth using their expertise to design the database in the first place.

The databases described in this chapter are quick to set up and affordable to buy for a small number of devices, but they do have limits for large teams and amounts of data. In such cases, you should consider more professional databases like Satellite Forms (www.satelliteforms.net). A computer professional can use this to quickly design a sophisticated user interface, including calculations that are triggered by the data you enter. This is how Dr Anatole Menon-Johansson designed a database to guide HIV therapy (www.vcpda.com). After filling out a long form about each patient's health and viral load, the clinician receives advice about the next appropriate prescription.

Clinical vignette of a GPs database

Dr Cochrane wanted to audit the small operations she carried out in her GP surgery. She bought HanDBase and downloaded a surgical logbook database. She entered each patient's details at the start of their operation. At followup appointments with the patient she would document any complications of that operation.

The data was backed up every time she synchronised her handheld computer. She could also view it on the desktop version of HanDBase and prepared audit reports for the practice's monthly management meeting.

Her partners were particularly impressed with the Personal Development Plan she downloaded for HanDBase. She used this to document every learning experience she had, including the lectures she attended and the PubMed searches she ran to find out information for her patients. She even documented the times that she beamed lecture notes to her colleagues as these counted as a teaching activity. At the end of the year she was proud at the amount of knowledge she could mention in her revalidation

▼ *Cont.*

forms but avoided the irritation that her colleagues felt at having to document the learning – it had been effortless to fill out the forms as she went about her education during the year.

She began designing her database for an audit of the practice's diabetes treatment. It was reasonably quick to design something usable but she knew that her design would not be perfect. After a few weeks of using the database she had gained enough experience to decide what data was most useful to gather, and what parts of the HanDBase interface would need to be speeded up for smooth data entry.

She applied for a grant through her Primary Care Trust to hire a Satellite Forms programmer. By showing him the HanDBase database she had already used and pointing out the areas of improvement that she needed he was able to create a professional product. Having paid for the work, the Trust was able to redistribute the software to all of the area's GPs and collect the data for epidemiological analysis.

11

Medical records

The ability to store patient records on a handheld computer is perhaps the feature that clinicians want the most, yet it also is perhaps the hardest to provide. If you are buying a device for yourself simply so that you can use it for medical records, then you should abandon the purchase and save your money.

Let me explain why I say this. From the previous chapter, you hopefully will have learnt that it is relatively easy to store information about your patients in your personal database. Buy HanDBase, create your forms and start entering patient data. The difficulty comes when you have to share information with other clinicians. Beaming may be enough for small teams, but for any more than five clinicians, you will need to synchronize your devices with a central computer...and that requires the help and support of the IT department.

The practice of medicine means that you almost always have to share information with your colleagues. Whether you do it in the paper notes or your institution's electronic medical records system, you must document what you do to the patients, so your team can provide appropriate care.

Thus if you decide that you do not want to share the patient notes on your device because of the complexity of involving the IT department, you will have to duplicate your writing: once for your device and again for the institution's notes. You will soon get tired of this, and we are all too busy to be duplicating work.

On the other hand, in institutions around the world, and increasingly with the support of national governments, IT departments are switching to electronic medical records. In many cases, handheld computers **are** part of that switch – or at least they are planned as the next stage. In such institutions, the doctors will be provided with handheld computers as part of good clinical care.

If you are in such an institution – congratulations, make use of your good fortune and enjoy your equipment!

If you are not, then you can change the institution and convince its decisions makers of the investment, but this is a long process and requires sustained effort. In the meantime, do not buy a handheld computer for yourself in the hope that you will get the support for medical records software. It will not come soon.

Of course, you should still buy the device for all the other advantages, and I hope that this book has convinced you of their value. The rest of this chapter will discuss the options you have as you move your institution to electronic medical records.

Medical records systems for individuals and small teams

The easiest way to begin managing your patient's records at the start is to buy software like Patient Tracker (www.patienttracker.com), which includes a handheld computer version and a PC version. This makes it easy to enter most of a patient's information at your clinic desk but to add more details with the handheld computer at the patient's home or to read those details on the device while away from your desk. The data is encrypted.

The software is designed for American clinicians and is ideal for small practices. It is not suitable for general practitioners in the UK, as more than 95% of their practices already have an electronic medical records system – and their complementary handheld computer versions are better. For doctors in hospitals in the UK that do not yet have such a system, however, Patient Tracker could be a useful purchase for each small team.

If for any reason you do not like Patient Tracker's interface, however, you cannot modify it. This is why so many clinicians like HanDBase, as each team can create the exact forms they need for their workflow. The effort of designing and implementing the forms is not trivial though and will take some time for experimentation.

Whatever you decide, one risk to think about is losing data. You can consider buying a backup SD card for your handheld computer from companies like MDM (www.gomdm.com) – for around $50, the card allows a complete backup of your device. Should you lose the data for any reason, you can restore it within a few minutes after inserting the card into the device. More dangerous is losing the device itself through theft or forgetfulness. This is why encryption is so important.

Bespoke medical records systems

With the financial and managerial support of your institution, you can consider a medical records system tailored to your team's needs. Scotland has wonderful examples of this, as the government has standardized data formats (which means that medical software designers can more easily share patient data between their products) and has provided budgets for software investments and target dates for implementation. Unlike the government in England, however, Scotland's government has not been involved in micromanaging implementation.

This has led to many new companies creating innovative products and tailoring them to clinicians' needs. For example, Extramed (www. extramed.co.uk) and Kelvin Connect (www.kelvinconnect.com) both created software that allowed hospital clinicians to read information on their patients during the ward round. The information is synchronized automatically between the handheld computer on the ward round, the PCs of the nurses in the medical assessment unit and the workstations of the radiologists in their offices.

What is interesting about these examples is the new working habits that they support and the planning that the team must go through. For example, in Lanarkshire, the software is a small part of the innovation of the night-time hospital emergency care teams. A small team of two nurses and five doctors triages and treats the hospital's inpatients overnight. In the morning, the nurses provide a report on each patient they treated, because it was the nurses that prescribed many of the drugs and the nurses that had the handheld computers.

For these habits, the doctors, nurses, managers and software developers worked together and decided on how best to proceed for their patients. When you understand the information in this book, you will be one of the best people in your institution to help guide the decision-making for handheld computers. Find out about the committees involved in such planning and contribute to them.

Off-the-shelf systems

Even if you cannot contribute to the design of a custom system for your team, you can still play an important role if your institution chooses an off-the-shelf medical records system. This is happening in England, where the government has designated specific medical records system providers for each region. Furthermore, in many institutions, including the practices of all general practitioners in England, complete medical records systems already exist. You will not be able to switch to a different provider, but you still can buy the handheld computer version of their software. For example Inchware (www.inchware.com) makes impressive PDA versions for the existing products of EMIS, iSoft, Torex and Vision in the UK, while IDX and McKesson in the US also have had their own mobile software for several years.

Even after the purchasing decision has been made, and even if the product is fixed and not customized, you still will play a crucial role. For example, you can take part in the early testing. This will mean that you can advise on the rate of deployment – which wards should come first – and will be ideally placed to provide training for your colleagues.

Such work is good for your career. For many clinicians, such satisfying work has prompted a switch to medical informatics as a specialty. In the end, of course, it will be the patients that benefit. Medical errors are many, expensive and dangerous. To reduce these and improve care governments around the world are investing billions of dollars in solutions. Electronic medical records are a vital part of these, and handheld computers are already making their mark. I hope that this book helps you bring the benefits to your patients.

Clinical vignette of medical records

Impressed by the work of Dr Cochrane in her general practice surgery, Dr Snow bought a handheld computer. It greatly improved his organization, and they designed a database to store audit information about their patients with diabetes for audits.

Soon, their seven colleagues wanted to make the same investment. In a practice meeting, they decided that each doctor should buy their own device to suit their tastes. Because the practice had an EMIS medical records system, the clinicians with Palm Powered devices could use the EMIS PDA software, while those with Pocket PCs could get EMIS-compatible PDA software from Inchware.

This allowed Dr Snow to take the records of the patients he would see on a home visit, refer to the prescriptions and past medical history while with the patient and make notes on the visit on the handheld computer. Once back in the practice, the new notes would synchronize back to the central computer and become available to the PCs and PDAs of the other doctors and nurses.

The software did not do everything the team required, however, so Dr Snow wrote a business case for the purchase of custom software to monitor the progress of patients with cardiological conditions and diabetes. He received funding from his primary care trust and found a small company in the area. They collaborated on the design of the software and made sure that it integrated into the existing EMIS system.

The product was so well suited to the management of the patients' conditions that he was able to coauthor several papers that documented the improved control of hypertension, and several practices in the surrounding area also invested in the software.

By this time, Dr Snow was hooked on the benefits of handheld computers for good clinical practice. He started a long-distance course in medical informatics, supported by a scholarship from his primary care trust, and searched for other areas in which he could improve patient care.

Index

N.B. Entries in **bold** denote PDA functions